THE ORTHODONTIC
ANSWER BOOK

THE ORTHODONTIC ANSWER BOOK

A Guide to the **Most Common Patient Questions**

JACK BURROW · BRITNEY WELCHEL · SAMUEL BURROW

DDS   DMD   DMD

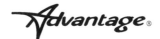

Published by Advantage, Charleston, South Carolina.
Member of Advantage Media Group.

ADVANTAGE is a registered trademark, and the Advantage colophon is a trademark of Advantage Media Group, Inc.

Printed in the United States of America.

10 9 8 7 6 5 4 3 2 1

ISBN: 978-1-64225-032-9
LCCN: 2018964071

Cover and layout design by: Wesley Strickland

This publication is designed to provide accurate and authoritative information in regard to the subject matter covered. It is sold with the understanding that the publisher is not engaged in rendering legal, accounting, or other professional services. If legal advice or other expert assistance is required, the services of a competent professional person should be sought.

 Advantage Media Group is proud to be a part of the Tree Neutral® program. Tree Neutral offsets the number of trees consumed in the production and printing of this book by taking proactive steps such as planting trees in direct proportion to the number of trees used to print books. To learn more about Tree Neutral, please visit **www.treeneutral.com**.

Advantage Media Group is a publisher of business, self-improvement, and professional development books and online learning. We help entrepreneurs, business leaders, and professionals share their Stories, Passion, and Knowledge to help others Learn & Grow. Do you have a manuscript or book idea that you would like us to consider for publishing? Please visit **advantagefamily.com** or call **1.866.775.1696**.

TABLE OF CONTENTS

PART I: BRACES—THE BASICS

PART II: SHOULD MY CHILD GET BRACES?

PART III: I'M IN BRACES BUT I HAVE QUESTIONS

PART VII: LIFE AFTER BRACES

PART VIII: CHOOSING A PROVIDER

CONCLUSION:

PREFACE

AS ORTHODONTISTS, WE KNOW there are a lot of options out there for straightening teeth and creating a beautiful smile. But there's also a lot of confusing information out there when it comes to orthodontics. How do you know where to turn?

Since orthodontic patients have a lot of questions—often the same ones—we put together this book of answers to the questions we hear most often. In the pages ahead, we hope to clarify some of the information about orthodontics to help you become more familiar with what orthodontics is about. We want you to see what sets us apart from other practices, that we are passionate about creating gorgeous smiles for patients, and that we strive to provide the highest level of individualized treatment. We want patients of all ages to become comfortable with the idea of undergoing treatment, because today, braces are not just for children and adolescents but also for adults.

This book is formatted a little differently than usual. The "chapters" are actually questions that people ask, and the content of each "chapter" is the answer to one of those questions. The book is meant to be a guidebook of sorts, designed for you to flip easily to the topic that interests you. And while we've included a lot of the questions and answers in the pages ahead, we are always happy to explain anything more in-depth, or answer any other questions not in this book.

Introduction

THE BURROW & WELCHEL DIFFERENCE

HELPING PATIENTS FEEL COMFORTABLE with treatment and achieve the smile of their dreams—that's what we like to call the "Burrow & Welchel difference."

That difference begins with a practice of unrivaled expertise and more than fifty years of combined experience. We are the only provider in our area with three board-certified orthodontists under one roof. Each of us has been through specific testing by the American Board of Orthodontics, certification that only about 30 percent of orthodontists go through. Board certification requires the orthodontist to demonstrate to their peers that they have the knowledge and skills to deliver the highest level of patient care. Certification is earned by passing a rigorous set of written, oral, and clinical exams, and must be renewed every ten years.

While training and experience are key to a good outcome in any orthodontic treatment, what really counts is that we work together as a team on every case. Instead of a single practitioner providing one-on-one treatment, at our practice it's really three-on-one. Every patient's case is reviewed by three sets of board-certified eyes as a means of quality assurance. Then we bring together our perspectives and collaborate on a comprehensive treatment plan.

1

Delivering multi-perspective care is possible through a unique level of seamless communication. We operate like a well-oiled machine when it comes to diagnosing and treating each patient's case. Yet we are approachable. Yes, our goal is to help you have a great smile, but we also want you to have a great experience while you're doing it.

While we have the expertise of a much larger practice, we are comfortably sized to make us accessible for any patient need. During treatment, we ensure that you have each doctor's cell phone number to give you a direct line should a need arise. No leaving a message on a machine. No going through an answering service. No waiting in a queue when calling in to the front desk. You're welcome to contact us directly with any issues or problems. Whether it's an emergency with your braces, a problem with the paying system, or any other issue, you have a direct line to the doctors providing care. We know that emergencies can disrupt your treatment—and your life—so we're willing to meet you any time outside of office hours to ensure that treatment continues as smoothly as possible.

As a family practice, we want to make patients feel like family, too. We treat patients as we would members of our own families, from performing a comprehensive initial exam to educating about treatment options to communicating every step of the way as they progress toward that smile they so desire. Having undergone our own orthodontic challenges, we know what it's like to be in the patient's shoes. So we go the extra mile to ensure that patients look forward to (and don't dread) each appointment. We want to ensure that patients know what to expect with every visit and with their role in treatment between appointments.

WHAT ELSE COMPRISES THE BURROW & WELCHEL DIFFERENCE?

For starters, we place an emphasis on the total health of your teeth. Straight teeth are great, but healthy teeth come first. We monitor hygiene at every appointment and work with patients to help them understand areas of improvement. We also know that function is crucial to a successful smile. Straighter teeth are easier to clean and maintain, which leads to healthier gums and healthier teeth in general. And in addition to lining up the teeth, our treatments are designed to correct the bite. We want to help the patient avoid irregular wear or chipping from upper and lower teeth that don't meet properly when biting down.

To ensure the most cosmetically pleasing, stable, and healthy smile, we create treatment plans that are customized to each patient's individual needs and wants. No two cases are the same. It all depends on the patient's skeletal, dental, and soft-tissue makeup. We look at the ideal position of each tooth and how it relates to the other teeth and to overall facial aesthetics. We don't just put on braces and straighten teeth. We want to ensure that the underlying structures of the face provide support for the lips and other facial features. We study each patient's teeth, jaws, and facial structure before creating a treatment plan that produces the desired end result and fits their lifestyle. We want to know what is going to work for you in terms of treatment options.

For instance, if you have a singular goal in mind—such as straightening one or two teeth or closing a gap—we may be able to accomplish that with what is known as limited treatment. This shortened treatment plan can fix a chief complaint without having to wear braces for years. However, with limited treatment, we still conduct a comprehensive evaluation to ensure that fixing one complaint won't lead to more complications. In cases like these, we typically offer multiple plans ranging from limited treatment to the ideal treatment (fixing all the issues we find as part of the evaluation). The consultation to discuss treatment includes education about any detrimental effects that can happen when fixing a single problem is not advisable.

Another Burrow & Welchel difference? Our modern offices and technology. We use state-of-the-art 3-D technologies for diagnosis and treatment. With 3-D technology, we are able to see where teeth are at the beginning of treatment and where we predict they will move during treatment. We can also determine how the movements of each tooth will affect other teeth, the soft tissues of the mouth, and the structures of the entire face.

Our technologies include digital intra-oral scanning, a "wand" that scans teeth to create a digital model. This scanner replaces the need for goopy impressions. The scan creates digital images that display on a computer screen and allow us to view and manipulate the teeth, helping us project movement throughout treatment. It is the latest in diagnosis and treatment planning.

Scanning technologies also include cone beam computed tomography (CBCT), which provides 3-D images of the jaws and teeth. CBCT images let us see beneath the soft tissues of the mouth to reveal issues such as impacted teeth or teeth that have yet to come in, or "erupt." With CBCT images, we can better diagnose patients and create more accurate and effective treatment plans.

In appliance therapy, we currently use metal twin braces and Clarity clear ceramic brackets. These, in our opinions, are the sturdiest brackets on the market. They both are very comfortable, very high technology brackets designed by 3M that allow us to do our work very efficiently. Along with the brackets, we use nickel-titanium wires that allow us to straighten teeth with slow, continuous forces that make movements a very gentle experience for patients. The wires also decrease the number of visits that patients make over the course of treatment.

We also offer straightening with both Invisalign and 3M Clarity clear aligners. And we offer Incognito lingual braces, which include brackets bonded to the backside of the teeth, making them virtually invisible from the front.

In auxiliary appliances, we are well versed in technologies such as skeletal plates, Herbst appliances, and temporary anchorage devices (TADs), all designed to help with complex movements.

As early testers for many companies that introduce products to the market, we get to see the latest technologies and provide feedback before the products hit the market to ensure that they are something we feel comfortable using on our patients.

While technology allows us to offer the latest advances in treatment, what really makes a difference with patients is being greeted by a friendly, supportive staff with years of experience working with children, teens, and adults. Something we can't teach is personality—that's why we hire people who are open and willing to answer questions and help us provide an excellent patient experience.

To ensure chair-side quality, every assistant goes through the Burrow & Welchel Training Academy before providing hands-on care. Academy training helps ensure that assistants treat according to our standards of care by first getting them up to speed with our orthodontics protocol, then progressing to training with manne-quins, followed by training on actual patients.

At Burrow & Welchel, we believe our practice is about more than providing orthodontic care. We feel our role also encompasses being an integral part of the communities we serve. To that end, we participate in fairly sizable community events each quarter, and every month, we give back in some way. For instance, we participate in organized events like TeamSmile's Carolina Panthers Day, where we provide free dental care to more than 250 children. Or we might sponsor a patient of ours who is a cancer survivor and is now running in a 5K race. One month we may hold a fun event in a school to educate kids on the value of good oral health, and another we may simply set up a booth at a fall festival and tie-dye T-shirts with kids. We're always looking for ways to creatively be out where we can get to know our neighbors and they can get to know us.

Like us so far? We think you'll like us even more after you see how enthusiastic we are about helping you have a great smile and a comfortable experience, and answering all your questions before and during the process. That's the Burrow & Welchel difference.

PART I

BRACES—THE BASICS

AREN'T ALL ORTHODONTISTS THE SAME?

When considering orthodontic treatment, it's important to understand as much as you can about your provider.

WHEN CHOOSING A provider for your orthodontic treatment, it's important to understand as much as you can. Since you or your child will be under that doctor's care for some time, you want someone you feel comfortable with—someone whose personality, training, and skills meet your needs.

All orthodontists are dentists; they start their training by completing dental school. But orthodontists go beyond that initial training with an additional two to three years of residency that includes hands-on patient care. In that specialty training, they learn not only about moving teeth for aesthetics, but also how to assess the bone structure and bite to ensure health along with a great smile.

While dentists and orthodontists both help patients have the best oral health, they focus on different aspects of that health. Dentists deal largely with the health of the teeth and gums. They typically provide services that deal with tooth decay and gum disease along with restorative services such as fillings, crowns, and bridges. They may even offer cosmetic options such as tooth whitening and veneers.

While some general dentists provide orthodontic treatment, it's important to understand that this is not their specialty. That's not what they do day in and day out.

Orthodontists also look at the health of the teeth and gums—a healthy mouth is crucial for the work that orthodontists do. However, orthodontists specialize in correcting the bite, straightening teeth, and ensuring that the structures of the mouth work well together. They have solutions for issues such as crowded teeth, overbite, underbite, or malaligned teeth.

While different orthodontists may offer the same or similar services, all orthodontists are not created equal. What sets us apart at Burrow & Welchel Orthodontics is that all three of our doctors have gone beyond the required training to practice as orthodontists. Each of us is board certified by the American Board of Orthodontics, a distinction that only about one in three orthodontists have achieved. Board certification requires an orthodontist to demonstrate to their peers, through a rigorous set of written, oral, and clinical exams, that they have the knowledge and skills to deliver the highest level of patient care.

We also hold ourselves to a higher standard through our commitment to continuing education, which keeps us up to date on the latest innovations and technology, and through our commitment to teaching current resident orthodontists. Dr. Samuel "Jack" Burrow III teaches at the University of North Carolina at Chapel Hill School of Dentistry; he and Dr. Samuel "Sam" Jackson Burrow IV have both lectured at Harvard University and at the Medical University of South Carolina; and Dr. Britney Welchel lectures at Baylor College of Dentistry. We also have the extra insight that comes from conducting research of our own.

WHAT ARE THE DIFFERENT TYPES OF BRACES?

There are different treatments depending on patient needs.

IN OUR PRACTICE, we use two types of braces to move teeth for orthodontic treatment: metal and ceramic. Both types of braces involve brackets that are bonded to the patient's teeth and connected by an archwire that applies gentle pressure to guide the teeth into alignment.

The metal braces we use are made of high-grade stainless steel. Today, these braces are smaller, more comfortable, and more attractive than braces of the past. Ceramic braces work the same as metal braces, but they are made of a translucent, ceramic material that blends with the tooth's natural color. Many patients choose ceramic brackets because they are barely noticeable on the teeth.

One concern that many patients have with the clear brackets is that they will discolor with time. Good news! The technology has evolved so much that the brackets remain beautifully clear for the duration of treatment. For this reason, many teens and adults tend to prefer the ceramic brackets. Yet, for those children who are excited about having bright braces colors on their teeth, there is still the option to have colorful alastics (also known as o-rings) around the clear brackets just as they can have on the metal brackets.

JACK BURROW · BRITNEY WELCHEL · SAMUEL BURROW

Bracket design varies between types and manufacturers. For instance, twin brackets require the colorful "o-ring" to engage the archwire, while self-ligating brackets use built-in doors to engage the archwire.

A commonly used self-ligating bracket is the Damon bracket. Whichever bracket is used, the most important point to remember is that teeth know no difference. Many research studies have analyzed the different bracket types, one of them conducted by Dr. Jack Burrow. All the research points to the same conclusion: Teeth feel a force, and that's what tells them to move. It really doesn't matter what type of bracket is used. What's more important is the experience of the doctor guiding treatment. As we always say: it's the chef that makes the meal, not the pan that they cook with.

Another option available for moving teeth is the Invisalign system, which is a series of clear aligners that are custom made to fit the teeth. Each aligner introduces a small amount of tooth movement as the patient progresses through treatment. Invisalign is a great option for many patients due to its many advantages. The aligners are removable, so there are no diet restrictions with Invisalign like there are with braces. You're able to eat all the sticky, chewy, gummy foods that you can't eat with braces. Additionally, the removable aspect of the aligners allows for ease of cleaning. You can brush like normal and there are no obstacles to floss around, allowing for a better oral hygiene environment.

Although Invisalign is ideal for people who want a low-maintenance option, not everyone is a good candidate for Invisalign. Invisalign only works when the aligners are worn, so people who aren't able to commit to wearing them the required twenty-one hours a day are not good candidates. While recent Invisalign enhancements have made it possible to treat more severe cases than in the past, very severe cases may still require metal braces as the best choice for moving teeth. Certain movements are just more predictable with braces. We are always willing to talk the pros and cons of each system and will make it clear which one we recommend to yield the safest, quickest, and most desirable outcome.

Invisalign Teen may be an option for the cosmetic-conscious teen—such as those in the local ballet troupe and those who are disciplined and will wear their aligners faithfully.

Some of the issues that orthodontic treatment and appliances (like braces) address include:

- **Underbite** occurs when the lower front teeth overlap the upper front teeth when the mouth is closed. Often, an underbite is caused by a lower jaw positioned too far forward.

- **Overjet** (commonly incorrectly referred to as "overbite") occurs when the upper front teeth are too forward or protrusive relative to the lower teeth. Often, an overjet is caused by a small lower jaw or when the jaw is set too far back.

- **Spacing** occurs when there are unattractive gaps between teeth.

- **Crowding** occurs when there is not enough space in the jaw for all the teeth.

- **Overbite**, also called a deep bite, occurs when there is excessive vertical overlap between the upper and lower front teeth with the mouth closed. Ideally, there should be a 25 percent overlap.

- **Open bite** occurs when there is a lack of vertical overlap between the upper and lower teeth when a person bites down.

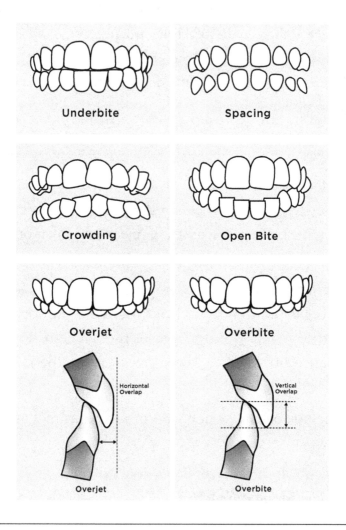

The length of time in braces or Invisalign is roughly the same and is customized to each patient's needs. However, with Invisalign, visits to the office occur less frequently. With braces, the patient must come in for an adjustment every eight to twelve weeks. Invisalign is more or less managed by the patient; visits to the office are only required every three to four months, since the orthodontist has pre-designed the movements into the patient's aligners. Of course, treatment time can also be affected by issues such as broken brackets, poor hygiene, or not following the doctor's orders.

HOW DOES INVISALIGN WORK?

Information about treatment with clear aligners.

THERE ARE MANY manufacturers of clear aligners; one well-known brand is Invisalign. The technology is a system of clear plastic aligners, or "trays," that are custom made for each patient. The patient progresses through a series of aligners as prescribed by the orthodontist, with each aligner providing a force that pushes the teeth in the desired direction. Just as with braces, the teeth feel a force that triggers them to move. In order to more efficiently express tooth movements, your orthodontist will bond attachments—basically tooth-colored buttons—to specific teeth to help move them in the desired directions. The attachments keep the aligners in place, and force applied perpendicular to the attachment by the aligner moves the tooth where it needs to go.

The process of Invisalign is simple. Once your orthodontist determines that clear aligner therapy is a good option for you, a digital 3-D scan is taken of your teeth. Gone are the days of "goopy" impressions. Instead, a wand is used to scan your teeth digitally and create a 3-D model. That 3-D model is sent to Invisalign virtually. The orthodontist then prescribes details such as the direction, velocity, and orientation they want the teeth to move. With those specifications, Invisalign creates a series of plastic aligners for the upper and lower sets of teeth. The number of aligners varies based on treatment complexity and the type of tooth movement being accomplished. Typically the patient changes to a new set of upper and lower aligners each week, which helps the aligners stay fresh and provide a continuous amount of tooth movement.

With Invisalign, teeth move at about the same speed as with braces. Each aligner allows for about a quarter millimeter of movement.

Roughly halfway through the treatment, the patient's progress is analyzed by the orthodontist and the treatment is fine-tuned through a refinement. In a refinement, the attachments are removed from the teeth, the teeth are scanned again, and additional aligners are made to new specifications.

There are some real plusses to using Invisalign for treatment. Invisalign requires less effort to maintain than bracket-and-wire braces. Since the aligners are removable, they can be taken out while eating. That means no restrictions on the types of foods a person can eat while being treated. The aligners are also removed for cleaning, so brushing and flossing don't require any extra effort. The aligners are transparent, so people often don't even notice that someone is wearing them. And since the patient switches the aligners out themselves, fewer visits to the orthodontist are needed for adjustments.

Invisalign has come a long way as a treatment for aligning teeth. Today, the aligners can work with certain growth modification appliances to treat even some complex cases, and some of the newest innovations can help posture the lower jaw forward in a growing child to correct an overbite. We may also make some difficult corrections first with other options, and then use Invisalign to finish the movements. For instance, we may first make a jaw correction with a palatal expander or put the patient in braces for a limited time just to correct a tooth that needs a significant amount of movement. Then we'll switch to Invisalign. That way, the majority of the movement is accomplished first, making the Invisalign part of treatment easier.

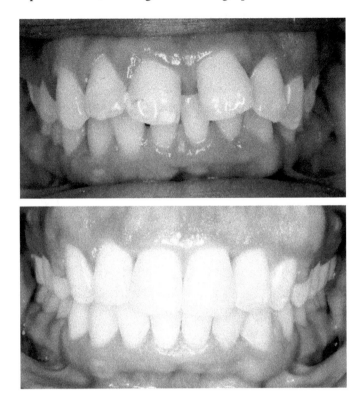

Before and after treatment using Invisalign.

Still, Invisalign is not for everyone. When a case involves a lot of movement or variables, we usually opt for braces because they are far more predictable. That's an advantage of being treated by an orthodontist, who understands the complexities of moving teeth. It's about more than just straightening teeth, it's about understanding what's needed in the way of tools and technique to treat even the most complex, intricate cases. As we like to say, it's the chef, not the pan, that makes a great meal.

There are many different brands of clear aligner therapy (SureSmile, ClearCorrect, 3M Clarity Aligners, and others).

Invisalign is just one that we currently use, and other types may be recommended for you depending on your treatment needs.

Again, as with all orthodontic technologies, it's not the appliance that fixes the dental problem. The orthodontist can use Invisalign or another brand of clear aligners as a means to help resolve a dental issue. It's like when you blow your nose with Kleenex. Everyone knows that brand, but it's just a tissue.

WHAT IF I JUST WANT ONE PROBLEM ADDRESSED?

Limited treatments are available for some cases.

SOME PEOPLE COME IN wanting help with teeth that are aesthetically unpleasing. They look in the mirror and see that a gap has developed in their front teeth, or they've got crowding in their lower teeth.

Often it's an adult who had braces when they were younger but didn't wear their retainers over time, so what they're seeing is a relapse—their teeth shifted after treatment. Since they wore braces before and know what treatment is about, they think getting their smile back is probably a quick fix.

In some cases, limited orthodontics can be done to simply align the anterior (front) teeth or fix a patient's chief complaint. This type of treatment applies gentle, light force to align teeth in as little as six months using tooth-colored brackets. It's actually a great option for adults who only need a few teeth corrected.

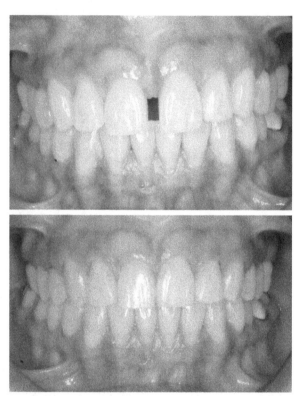

This patient presented to BWO with concerns only for upper spacing. Limited upper treatment was completed in six months, resulting in a beautiful, cosmetic outcome.

However, before we offer limited treatment, we diagnose each patient individually and form a specific treatment plan. If limited treatment is an option, it is offered among other alternatives ranging from limited to ideal. Certainly, some patients have a fantastic bite and all they really need is a couple of teeth realigned. And that may only take six to eight months of clear aligners or braces.

But if a patient's bite doesn't fit together correctly, or if moving teeth will change the bite and cause problems, we'll recommend comprehensive treatment. Otherwise, for example, moving the teeth on the upper jaw without moving teeth on the lower jaw could change your bite, and if your bite doesn't fit it could cause muscle irritation, which could cause joint problems. In other words, correcting what looks like a minor problem could lead to a cascade of issues.

Here again, it's best to see a certified orthodontist, who can accurately predict the outcome of moving even a few teeth.

CAN ORTHODONTICS HELP WITH MY SLEEP APNEA?

Sleep issues often require a multidisciplinary approach.

SLEEP APNEA, OR obstructive sleep apnea (OSA), is defined as cessation or interruption of normal breathing. Common symptoms of sleep apnea include snoring, disruption of sleep from constantly waking up gasping for breath, and daytime fatigue.

In children, sleep apnea symptoms may have the same characteristics as attention-deficit/hyperactivity disorder, or ADHD. Children who are hyperactive or who struggle to keep up in school may be diagnosed as having ADHD when the reality is that they're suffering from obstructive sleep apnea issues that have gone undiagnosed—they're just tired and can't pay attention.

OSA often is the result of an obstruction in the airway, anywhere from the tip of the nose to the throat. In children, that obstruction may be caused in part by enlarged tonsils and adenoids. While surgical removal of the tonsils and adenoids may alleviate some of the child's symptoms, they may still have an obstruction somewhere else in their airway.

When we see children for an orthodontic evaluation—as early as age seven, as recommended by the American Association of Orthodontists—we also talk to the parents about some of the signs of sleep apnea. Does the child snore during sleep? Are there any noticeable breathing problems? Does the child have trouble staying awake or paying attention in school?

We also look for signs that may indicate the potential for breathing problems, such as an unstable bite or a narrow upper jaw. If we see signs, we use radiography (X-rays) to thoroughly assess the airway. That helps us determine whether their situation warrants a referral to an ear, nose, and throat specialist (ENT), or whether it's something we want to watch as part of our ongoing monitoring of the child's growth.

If the child is diagnosed as having sleep apnea, then one of the orthodontic treatments that might be considered includes using a palatal expander. A palatal expander is an appliance that fits inside the roof of the child's mouth to widen the upper jaw. That's possible in youth because there is a suture that runs from front to back in the roof of the mouth. Early in life, that suture is made of fibrous tissue. By a certain age, that material fuses together and becomes bone. Until it fuses, the suture can be widened. Since the roof of the mouth is the floor of the nose, the expander may also help to widen the nasal airway.[1] However, a recent study has found that while palatal expanders work well to widen the upper jaw—which is ideal for fixing the bite—there is no scientific evidence to prove the effectiveness of expansion in treating sleep apnea.[2] What works great

---

1   Di Carlo, Gabriele, et al., "Rapid Maxillary Expansion and Upper Airway Morphology: A Systematic Review on the Role of Cone Beam Computed Tomography," BioMed Research International, July 16, 2017, https://www.ncbi.nlm.nih.gov/pmc/articles/PMC5534278/.

2   Ying Zhao et al., "Oropharyngeal airway changes after rapid palatal expansion evaluated with cone-beam computed tomography," AJO-DO 137, no. 4 (April 2010): S71–S78, https://10.1016/j.ajodo.2008.08.026.

in one child may only mean slight improvement in another, and no improvement in another.

So, when we see signs of potential sleep apnea, whether we treat with an expander appliance or not, we always refer the child to an ENT for an evaluation and a sleep study.

Similarly, when it comes to adults and sleep apnea, we typically take a multidisciplinary approach. The symptoms in adults are nearly the same as in children: snoring, waking from sleep, daytime fatigue, and lack of mental clarity. In adults, however, sleep apnea can actually lead to more severe health problems such as hypertension.

Treatment for adults usually includes a referral to an oral surgeon, who will have the patient undergo a sleep study. Depending on the diagnosis, orthodontic treatments may involve braces to set the jaw up for orthognathic surgery (jaw surgery), which work together to align the teeth and open up the airway. There are also oral appliances that can be worn at night to help open the airway during sleep. These shift the lower jaw forward to open the airway for people with mild cases of sleep apnea but are typically not indicated as long-term solutions for sleep apnea, as dental side effects can occur with prolonged use.

WHAT ORTHODONTIC TREATMENTS ADDRESS "TMJ"?

Orthodontics and problems of the temporomandibular joint—the jaw joint.

PATIENTS OFTEN TELL US they have "TMJ," a term often used mistakenly when referring to TMD, a disorder of the TMJ—the temporomandibular joint, or jaw joint. Symptoms of TMD commonly include pain or tenderness in the jaw or jaw joint area, pain when chewing, a popping noise in the jaw joint, facial pain and headaches, and difficulty opening and closing the mouth, sometimes to the point of the jaw locking.

The good news is that treating TMD doesn't have to be invasive. TMD can occur as a result of the muscles of the jaw joint or the joint itself. Most of the cases that we see involve muscular issues stemming from the patient clenching and grinding their teeth while sleeping— imagine the pressure you're putting on the structures of your face if you're clenching and grinding your teeth all night. For these patients, we can create a night guard that is fitted to the teeth and worn during sleep to take the pressure off the muscles and help prevent them from tensing up. Muscle relaxers can also help when a person is under a lot of stress, which is one reason people clench and grind their teeth at night. When the joint is the culprit—usually damaged from internal issues such as bone degeneration or external forces such as a blow to the face—the bite may be affected. With braces, we can correct the bite, and that may give some relief for TMD. But that's not always the case.

To diagnose TMD, we start by looking at the actual TMJ in a patient's radiograph (X-ray). Often, that lets us see whether there are any degenerative joint issues—if the condyle, or the end of the jaw bone, is worn down, that tells us there is some damage to the joint. If that's the case, we often refer the patient out for an MRI and potentially a consult with an oral surgeon. If we don't see damage, we suspect the issue is more muscular. At that point, we ask questions to find out if, for instance, a spouse has witnessed clenching and grinding. We also look for wear patterns on the teeth that show us clinically whether the patient is grinding their teeth all night.

The bottom line with TMD is that it can be difficult to diagnose, and the symptoms and treatment can vary from patient to patient. A treatment that may significantly reduce pain for one patient may do nothing for someone else. For instance, braces may correct the bite in one patient and alleviate some of the pain of their TMD. But in another patient, the braces may correct their bite but not the TMD pain.

That's why with TMD, we try to determine the source of the problem before treatment starts. And since multiple factors can be the culprit, treating TMD often requires several treatments to finally get some relief.

PART II:

SHOULD MY CHILD GET BRACES?

WHEN WILL MY CHILD BE READY FOR ORTHODONTIC TREATMENT?

Children as young as age seven should be evaluated to head off developmental problems.

THE AMERICAN ASSOCIATION of Orthodontists recommends children see an orthodontist by age seven. At that age, we evaluate the child to determine if the teeth, jaws, and facial structures have any issues that need to be addressed while the child is developing.

No two mouths are the same. Each has its own ideal in the way of balance and harmony—that's what we're looking for in that first exam in these key areas: the soft tissue, teeth, and jaws, and then all other structures, including the airway.

Orthodontists not only have the ability to move teeth, but we can also influence the way the soft tissue drapes over the teeth, thus providing balance to the profile. If, for instance, a change in lip or chin position is desired, treatment mechanics will be properly applied to achieve these goals. Next, we analyze the teeth themselves. At the initial consultation, we look to see how the teeth are erupting: Are they coming in symmetrically and in the proper sequence? Are there any missing or extra teeth? Is there enough room for all the teeth? Then we look at the skeletal component. With the jaws, we're looking at the relation of the upper and lower jaws to each other and to the overall skull. We're also looking at the width of the upper jaw—a narrow upper jaw can cause all kinds of problems down the road, and expanding it is best done at a very young age. Lastly, we look at miscellaneous issues such as the airway, which can affect the child's development.

The goal of treating a child at age seven, often known as Phase I or early intervention treatment, is essentially to ensure that the foundation is developing correctly. The finishing touches come later, in what's known as Phase II treatment, after all or most of the adult teeth have come in. In girls, that is usually around age eleven; in boys, around age twelve.

Often Phase I treatment involves expanding the upper jaw to widen it and align its shape with the lower jaw. Expansion can also be done later, during Phase II treatment, also known as comprehensive orthodontics. One reason to do expansion in Phase I is to prevent asymmetric jaw growth, which can occur if a child has functional issues with their jaws that are causing them to shift their bite.

Some issues are best addressed in Phase I, others in Phase II. Here are the problems we may address early in a child's development:

- **Significant underbite**. If the bite doesn't match because of a significant underbite, where the lower teeth are more forward than the upper teeth, then we want to start treatment early. An underbite can be due to the jaw relationship, where the lower jaw is more prominent than the upper jaw, or it can be due to tooth position, where the top teeth tilt in behind the lower teeth. An underbite can occur with a single tooth or multiple teeth.

  Sometimes the underbite can involve a combination of both a jaw issue and tilted teeth. As part of our diagnosis, we determine the cause of the underbite to see whether it's an issue that can be treated with braces alone or whether it also needs an orthopedic correction—a change in the jaw structure. If the underbite is the result of flared teeth, it's because of the way the teeth erupted—for instance, a single tooth is usually a dental issue that can be corrected with braces. But typically, an underbite is a jaw structural issue that requires correction in the form of a face mask—headgear that helps pull the jaw forward. We also use what are known as skeletal plates, which are plated onto the bone on the top jaw toward the back of the mouth, and on the bottom jaw toward the front. These plates are accompanied by elastics to help accelerate the growth of the upper jaw and restrict the growth of the lower jaw. They can often prevent the need for a surgical procedure in the future. Dr. Jack Burrow was one of the first practitioners to use skeletal plates for early correction. He first used them more than twenty years ago while teaching at the University of North Carolina, and he has continued to build on his experience in using them to correct the bite early and prevent the invasive surgery needed after growth.

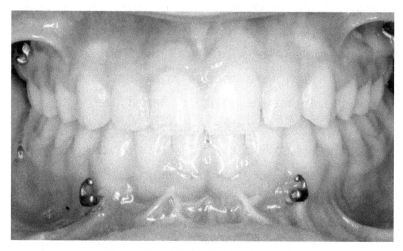

Example of Class III Skeletal Plates.

With certain bites, especially underbites, we ask about family history to determine whether there is a strong genetic connection. That helps with decisions about treatment. For instance, if dad had a significant underbite, we may delay treatment until we observe how strong the family resemblance is. If there's too much correction needed for orthodontic treatment alone, then jaw surgery will likely be needed at some point.

- **Crossbite**. There are different types of crossbites. In an ideal bite, the upper jaw should be a little wider than the lower jaw; the teeth in the upper arch of the jaw should be situated outside the lower teeth, like the lid to a shoebox. A posterior crossbite occurs when the upper jaw is too narrow, so that the top teeth at the back of the mouth are situated slightly on the inside of the bottom teeth. An anterior crossbite is one in which the lower teeth in the front are outside the upper teeth—an underbite is an example of an anterior crossbite. A unilateral crossbite is a crossbite on only one side of the mouth, while a bilateral crossbite involves both sides.

- **Open bite**. In an ideal situation, the upper front teeth overlap the lower front teeth by about 25 percent. When the front teeth are erupting, there is a natural open bite, with a bit of a gap between the upper and lower teeth. Unfortunately, in the early years, a child can develop habits such as thumb sucking, inadequate tongue posture, or airway issues that can worsen that gap and create problems that are more difficult to correct later on. If we can intervene early enough and correct those habits, the teeth will naturally grow together as they should. If we don't correct those habits, or we don't see a patient until later as a teen when their adult teeth are in and their jaws are skeletally mature, then correcting that open bite is more involved. At that point, it requires stopping the habit in combination with orthodontic treatment.

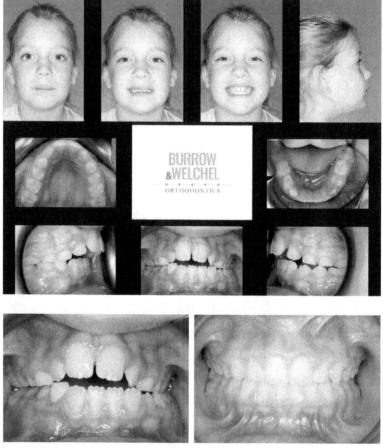

Phase I. treatment for open bite closure with thumb habit appliance and expander, followed by Phase II for overjet correction.

- **Thumb-sucking habits** can alter a child's bite and lead to an open bite. Typically, correcting this habit starts by discussing the problem with the patient and parent to make them aware of how detrimental thumb sucking is to the bite. If the child fails to stop the habit on their own, the next step may be to treat with a habit appliance, which is affixed to the teeth and prevents the child from inserting their thumb into their mouth.

- **Tongue posture**. The tongue is one of the body's strongest muscles. When it functions or rests incorrectly—such as pushing through the front teeth during a swallow or as a force of habit because of some other malformation in the mouth—the tongue can cause an open bite. For this condition, we refer the patient to a myofunctional therapist to retrain the tongue to behave as it should. By correcting the function of the tongue in Phase I treatment, we don't have to address the problems it causes when we get to Phase II.

- **Obstructed airway**. An obstruction of the airway can potentially alter a child's development—a child who can't breathe well can suffer all sorts of problems, from sleep disruptions to attention disorders.

- **Congenital craniofacial anomalies**. Children with Down syndrome and certain craniofacial syndromes can have systemic issues such as cleft lip and palate or extreme discrepancy in the position of the jaws. Depending on the situation, we may work with oral or plastic surgeons to address these issues. With these children, it usually takes a multidisciplinary team approach to resolve the problems they are having.

- **Congenitally missing teeth**. In very young children, the most common missing teeth we find are the wisdom teeth and the upper lateral incisors—the second tooth from the middle of the front. While it's generally a good thing to be missing wisdom teeth, it's usually best to replace the upper lateral incisors in some way. Replacing one of these involves either an implant or moving the canine tooth into the space to substitute for that missing tooth. By seeing the child early, we're able to start formulating a plan as to which direction we're going to go with treatment. Typically, filling the space occurs in Phase II, when all the adult teeth are in.

- **Anterior-posterior discrepancies** are big discrepancies in the forward to back position of the jaw. For instance, an overjet occurs when the front teeth are positioned forward a lot farther than the bottom teeth. That may be caused by the position of the teeth or the jaws.

- **Vertical bite discrepancies**. An overbite is the vertical overlap of the teeth, which ideally is only about 25 percent. A deep bite, or excessive overbite, is anything beyond that—a bite so extreme that the lower teeth can actually impinge on the palate.

- **Cosmetic treatment**. Often a parent will come in and tell us they just want braces on their child's front teeth for cosmetic purposes, even if Phase I is not needed. Their child is being bullied, they explain, so they're looking for a quick fix. Often it's because a child's front teeth are sticking out too far because of the way their jaws are positioned or from a thumb- or lip-sucking habit. Those forward teeth are not something we would normally fix in Phase I. But a six-month treatment of braces on a few select teeth can certainly change a child's life during those formative years while they're in late elementary or early middle school and waiting for comprehensive orthodontics. Often we'll do that just for the aesthetics and social aspect.

We take a conservative approach to Phase I treatment, only addressing issues that take advantage of that early growth or those that can cause long-term problems if left untreated. If problems are identified, treatment often waits another year or two to allow for that additional growth and to allow the child to get comfortable with us and with the treatment. Usually, all four of the front adult teeth and the six-year molars in the back should be in place before Phase I treatment begins. Phase I treatment typically lasts about twelve months, and then the results are retained until Phase II treatment begins.

Most children we see don't need any treatment at that early age of seven. For those who don't need treatment, we monitor their progress on an annual basis with complimentary appointments. We want to ensure that everything is developing as it should, or in a way that will allow treatment later on, when all the adult teeth are in. Those visits also allow the child to meet and get comfortable with the orthodontist, to build a relationship for the future when treatment may be needed.

Undergoing Phase I treatment does not prevent a need for treatment in Phase II. In fact, most patients who undergo Phase I to correct foundational issues also need Phase II treatment later as an adolescent, to ensure that all the teeth are aligned together. Phase I treatment does not shorten the amount of time in Phase II, but it can prevent problems from getting worse and can improve the ability to treat any complications that arise between the phases.

DOES MY CHILD REALLY NEED BRACES?

There are three types of issues that can be addressed with braces: aesthetics, phonetics, and function.

YES, BRACES CAN HELP create a pleasing smile. But treatment with braces can also help correct speech issues and problems affecting the function of the mouth. Those are the three types of issues we can address with braces: aesthetics, phonetics, and function.

Left untreated, problems in the mouth can worsen over time. Now, no one ever died from an overbite—if your teeth have always been in a certain position, then that's normal to you. But with braces, you will notice a change in your bite: it's easier to eat when your teeth are aligned—easier to bite into a sandwich, easier to eat fine foods like lettuce.

Here are some of the reasons to consider braces and some of the issues that braces can correct:

AESTHETICS—CROWDING/CROOKED TEETH

Teeth crowd and become crooked for a number of reasons. When there isn't enough room in the jawbone for all the teeth, they can crowd while erupting or coming in.

Teeth can also crowd if they are not retained after orthodontic treatment. Oftentimes, the amount of crowding can be so severe that extractions of premolars may be necessary for all teeth to properly align and maintain their ideal angulation.

There are multiple surges in tooth movement throughout life. One of those surges occurs at roughly the same time that the wisdom teeth start to come in. That makes people want to point to the eruption of wisdom teeth as the reason for their teeth moving and growing crooked, but the two events are actually not related. Molars don't necessarily dictate whether teeth will become crowded. Teeth can crowd even in those patients who do not have wisdom teeth. And they almost surely will crowd if retainers aren't worn following treatment.

Just as other parts of the body change over time—your hair changes, your skin changes—teeth are no different. Teeth move with time. But by having orthodontic treatment at a young age and then wearing a retainer, they can stay in position for the long term.

Not only is crowding less attractive, but crowded teeth can also be less healthy. Straight teeth are easier to clean, which decreases the chances of developing cavities and periodontal or gum disease. Left untreated, cavities can become much bigger problems and, like gum disease, can ultimately lead to bone loss and even tooth loss. That can potentially be prevented by simply having the teeth aligned, making them easy to clean and less susceptible to cavities and gum disease.

There are also social and emotional aspects to crooked teeth. Quality of life is better: Children with crooked teeth are often bullied. Adults with straight teeth are more likely to be hired, and to be successful overall.[3]

---

3   John Roger Feusier, "Does orthodontic treatment in adolescents affect quality of life? A practice-based research model," Graduate thesis, submitted to the Office of Graduate and Professional Studies of Texas A&M University, May 2015.

PHONETICS—SPEECH PROBLEMS

There's a certain position that the upper incisors need to be in so that the lip and the tongue and the teeth work in unison to provide the "s" and "th" sounds. If the front teeth, for example, are really tilted or positioned forward, it's difficult to articulate well by placing the tongue where it needs to be on the teeth. Braces can help correct the teeth and jaw positions so that the patient can articulate better.

FUNCTION—ALIGNING THE BITE, IDENTIFYING AIRWAY ISSUES

A well-aligned bite can prevent unnecessary damage to the teeth. When the bite is uneven—as with an underbite, overbite, crossbite, and other malformations—the teeth can begin to wear unevenly. In some situations, even the enamel can be worn away—and once that enamel is gone, it's gone forever. So, putting the teeth in the proper position can prevent long-term wear of the teeth. An improper bite can even cause an excessive load on one side of the joint versus the other, asymmetry that can begin to cause issues such as broken, cracked, or chipped teeth, as well as temporomandibular disorder (TMD), a disorder of the temporomandibular joint, or jaw joint.

An uneven bite can also lead to bruxing. Bruxing is a habit of clenching and grinding—usually during sleep or in times of great stress—that can cause considerable damage to teeth. There are a number of reasons why people brux, and there is no guarantee that braces will correct bruxing. Children often brux, but they tend to grow out of the habit. However, when bruxing is caused by premature contact—for instance, one tooth is longer than the others and is the first to contact during a bite—it can ultimately cause a person to brux subconsciously to try to get the teeth in a better position. Using braces can align the bite to correct that premature contact. But for bruxers, we typically also recommend a night guard or splint therapy.

Studies show that appliance therapy to reshape the upper jaw and expand the roof of the mouth can also help open the nasal airway in some patients. With airway issues, we take a very conservative approach to treatment and often refer the patient to other specialists. In the most extreme cases—patients who have severe sleep apnea— treatment for airway issues may include tonsil and adenoid removal or braces in combination with jaw surgery to move the lower and even the upper jaw forward.

With the 3-D images produced by cone beam computed tomography (CBCT)—basically an X-ray scanner—we can analyze whether there's any sort of obstruction in the nasal passages or the throat. If we see enlarged adenoids or tonsils, for instance, we may refer the child to an ear, nose, and throat specialist (ENT) for a consult.

With children, we recommend an initial consultation at age seven to look for any issues that may affect development. If no treatment is recommended at that time, we monitor the child until the adult teeth are in, at which point we may recommend other treatments. Fortunately, only a low percentage of children seen at age seven are in need of early orthodontic treatment.

PART III:

I'M IN BRACES BUT I HAVE QUESTIONS

HOW LONG DO I HAVE TO WEAR BRACES?

Orthodontic needs are determined largely by biology.

EVERY PATIENT'S ORTHODONTIC needs are a little different and are determined largely by biology. Applying the same force to moving teeth on two different patients will have different effects. While one patient may experience pain very quickly and very acutely, another patient may feel no pain at all. Similarly, while one patient's teeth may move very quickly, another patient's teeth may move slower; that rate of movement can determine when treatment is complete.

Our practice is very research oriented; we take a scientific approach to customizing treatment to each patient's need. By understanding the biology behind the movement of teeth, we can come up with average ranges that apply to most cases. For instance, the average for full orthodontic treatment tends to be eighteen to twenty-four months. Once we see the patient, however, and diagnose the issues they are having, we can more accurately project the length of time that treatment is expected to take. By getting to the root of the problem and creating a treatment plan, we can gauge an average treatment time.

Remember, it's not the braces that move teeth, it's the doctor guiding the braces. As a case in point, despite big claims being made about self-ligating brackets moving teeth faster, there are innumerable studies that prove otherwise. A lot of salesmanship recently has been put into marketing these brackets, but the bracket is certainly not going to determine treatment time. What matters is the biology of the patient and the experience and expertise of the orthodontist guiding treatment. It's more the practitioner's hand and how he or she sets up diagnosis and treatment that determines the treatment time. Biologically, on average, teeth can only move one millimeter per month. And in reality, the more force placed on a tooth, the less it's going to move. This is due to "undermining resorption," whereby the blood vessels surrounding the tooth are obstructed, thus decreasing cells in that area for the inflammatory response and restricting movement of the tooth.

Again, it's all about proper diagnosis and dedication to treatment. Think of it this way: When you dine at a nice restaurant and enjoy your meal, you don't typically ask about the brand of cookware the chef used. You're more interested in the recipe itself and the techniques of the chef: the ingredients, what temperatures were used, any special methods for preparing the food. But you're not going to ask for the name of the knife or the maker of the sauté pan.

With orthodontics, the teeth don't care what type of bracket they have on. They care what type of force and angulation are placed on them by the wire and the bracket. Since orthodontists use the same wires and the same appliances to move teeth, the proof is in the outcomes.

Something that has changed over time is the average treatment time between visits. Today, braces only require visits every eight to ten weeks. Parents who had braces as a child often expect that braces will require visits every four to six weeks. But because of the nickel-titanium wires and the progression in some of the appliances today from where they were, the time between appointments is longer.

With Invisalign—the clear aligners that are one form of treatment used to straighten teeth and correct other problems—even fewer visits are required. In some cases, visits can be spaced as much as sixteen or eighteen weeks apart.

While each case comes with estimated treatment times, there are factors that can affect treatment. The truth is, with treatment, we see patients about every eight weeks or so, but during all that in-between time, it's up to the patient to be proactive in taking care of their braces as agreed to as part of the treatment plan.

Factors that can affect treatment times include broken brackets, poor hygiene, and noncompliance with components like elastics. You can imagine how something like broken brackets can disrupt treatment time: If you can't get to the office for a couple of days, you're losing time that the brackets could be moving teeth. If, as a patient, you're lax about using the elastics as prescribed, or if you fail to brush your teeth and end up with gum disease or tooth decay, that can delay treatment for months. Teeth move much better in an oral environment that's clean and healthy, because the cells are able to do their job as opposed to being interfered with by inflammation.

There are two types of cells in the body that move teeth: osteoclasts and osteoblasts. The teeth live in the bones of the jaws. When we put pressure on a tooth, osteoclasts in the direction in which the tooth is moving break down the bone to allow space for the tooth to move. As the tooth moves into the new space, osteoblasts come in behind the tooth and fill the space the tooth just left. So teeth stay very active in the bone during orthodontic treatment. But if inflammation sets in because of poor hygiene—insufficient brushing and flossing—then the osteoclasts and osteoblasts struggle to do their job. That can affect the movement of the teeth.

That's the reason treatment is customized: each patient's case is based on their needs, wants, habits, and biology.

REALLY? NO POPCORN
WHILE WEARING BRACES?

Patient commitment to caring for braces helps achieve a successful outcome.

WHEN WE PLACE braces on a patient, we tell them we're putting something on their teeth that is not naturally supposed to be there. That's especially important for patients who have never worn braces to know. While the brackets for the braces are bonded to the teeth with a strong adhesive, we also want those braces to come off at some point in time, so it's a bit of a balancing act determining how well we bond the brackets to the teeth. We want the brackets to hold, but we also want them to release at the end of treatment.

But it's not solely up to the orthodontist to determine whether braces stay put. It also takes a commitment on behalf of the patient to get a successful outcome. That includes a change in lifestyle for the duration of treatment.

Lifestyle changes include considering the types of food you eat. Some foods require some modification when eating; others may be best to avoid altogether until the braces come off. For instance, crunchy foods like raw carrot sticks can be eaten if they are cut up in bite-size pieces. Apples can be cut into slices. With foods like these, however, it's best to be mindful—if it feels like there is excess pressure on the bracket, the bracket may be on the verge of breaking. Eating cooked carrots may be a better option while in braces. And with corn on the cob, for example, simply remove the corn from the cob before eating.

Popcorn is one food that is best to eat with care or avoid altogether. While the popped corn itself is soft enough to eat, unpopped kernels are hard and can break a bracket loose from the teeth. Husks can also get caught in the braces and can be difficult to clean out of teeth. Having that food on the tooth for any length of time can cause bacteria problems. Popcorn can be removed from the restrictions list if you prove that you can have good oral hygiene and for as long as you can keep that up.

During a treatment consultation, we will go over a complete list of food items that you should refrain from eating while in braces. They include ice, hard candy, and sticky foods such as caramel, taffy, and gum. Keeping these out of your diet will be healthier for your teeth and prevent your braces from being damaged.

In addition to watching the foods you eat, braces take a bit of extra care when it comes to cleaning. When we place braces on the teeth, we're adding surface area to the tooth, additional places where food can collect. Without regular brushing, the bacteria that normally protects the mouth feeds on the carbohydrates and other foods left on the teeth. Bacteria secrete acid, and that acid breaks down the enamel. Broken down enamel causes scarring of the teeth. Maybe you've seen those white spots on teeth after braces were removed? That's not from the braces themselves, those white spots are the scarring that comes from leaving food on the teeth for bacteria to feed on.

That's why it's important to get the food and sugar off the teeth after eating. We recommend brushing and flossing after meals, because the longer the food sits on the teeth, the more bacteria can build up and feed. We also recommend avoiding sipping on sugary sodas or fruit drinks all day long. Without cleaning the teeth, that sugar just builds up on the teeth and creates an acidic environment. If soda or fruit juices are a must, we recommend having them with a meal, and then brushing and flossing after that meal.

With kids, we typically tell them to brush and floss for two minutes after breakfast but not to worry about brushing and flossing at school. Instead, we want them to have a good, two-minute brushing when they get home, and then a four-minute brushing and flossing before bedtime. With adults, we recommend brushing and flossing three times a day, and then flossing and using a proxy brush right before bedtime. A proxy brush is a small brush that gets up under the wire.

Flossing is also a bit more challenging with braces. We show patients how to use what's known as "super floss," which is a floss with built-in threaders to help guide the floss around the wires and between the teeth.

A water flosser, such as a Waterpik, is also a good tool for cleaning and flossing because it breaks up food and plaque that might be on the teeth. However, a water flosser does not replace brushing and flossing, it's just an add-on to your overall hygiene success. Brushing will do half the work, the proxy brush will get another 10 percent of the cleaning done, and flossing will take care of the rest.

Patients are given reminders and encouragement with each visit to help them understand whether they're on track with their hygiene or whether there are areas that are being missed with brushing and flossing. The goal is to keep teeth and gums clean and healthy to avoid inflammation or infections in the mouth, as these can delay treatment.

Our practice provides an additional level of protection from bacteria during the bonding process. If you are a candidate for it, a sealant can be placed to act as a shield over the entire surface of the tooth enamel, thus protecting it from white spot lesions and/or decay. In addition, a fluoridated toothpaste is prescribed to continually activate the sealant and provide additional mineralization to the tooth.

As expected, we encourage and require patients to continue six-month cleaning appointments with their dentist. Often, if hygiene needs additional attention, a three-month cleaning appointment interval may be recommended.

WILL I HAVE TO WEAR HEADGEAR?

Technologies today make braces a far better experience.

ORTHODONTICS IS ONE industry that has seen significant advances over the years. Often, parents of our younger patients had braces when they were young—treatment that, for most, did not instill fond memories.

While the goals of treatment are still very similar—orthodontics straightens teeth and corrects the bite—the technologies that we use today make treatment a far better experience overall.

For instance, one of the most dreaded parts of treatment in the past involved wearing headgear—a device that attached to the braces and was worn outside the head. The headgear was designed to use the skull as leverage to hold back the upper jaw in order to let the lower jaw catch up in growth. Today, a modern version of headgear is used in rare cases where the patient has a very pronounced upper jaw. But we have better technologies that can accomplish special movements; these adjunct appliances are worn inside the mouth to correct jaw malformations.

Here are some of the technologies we use today that make treatment easier on the patient.

HERBST APPLIANCE

The Herbst appliance is used to help the lower jaw grow forward to match it to the upper jaw. It has a similar effect as headgear, but rather than just hold back the upper jaw while waiting for the lower jaw to grow forward, the Herbst can accelerate growth of the lower jaw while restricting growth of the upper jaw, thus providing time for the deficient lower jaw to "catch up" with the upper.

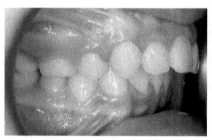 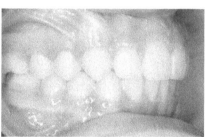

Before treatment with the Herbst appliance. Note the position of the mandibular canine relative to the maxillary canine (class II malocclusion).

After treatment with the Herbst appliance. The overjet has been resolved and the canines are now in class I position.

The appliance consists of a bar that is attached to the braces, from upper to lower molar, and worn inside the mouth. Although it's a bit cumbersome at first, the results that it produces are incredible. When we evaluate a patient, we determine whether the Herbst is a good choice for treatment. The Herbst is a great solution that can prevent the patient from having to undergo jaw surgery.

And compliance is no problem with the Herbst. The only extra care needed is the same as with braces—just take care with what you eat and drink and keep the appliance clean with regular brushing.

TEMPORARY ANCHORAGE DEVICES (TADS)

TADs are simple anchorage devices that are placed in the mouth to allow us to correct a dental issue without the use of adjunct appliances such as a headgear.

TADs allow us to use forces in ways we weren't able to in the past. TADs are small, screw-like implants used to provide a stable anchorage point about which to move teeth. In physics, for every force there's an opposite and equal force. Oftentimes, we don't want to provide a reciprocal force on a tooth. So planning has to take into account those inverted forces. With TADs, we can put force on a specific tooth or group of teeth, and it will move as we need it to without also applying negative force to another tooth. This works because the TAD is screwed into the alveolar or extra-alveolar bone and used as an anchorage point and tied to a specific tooth without affecting others. TADs are so much more efficient, and they allow us to do movements that beforehand were a lot harder, if not impossible to do.

Before   *During*

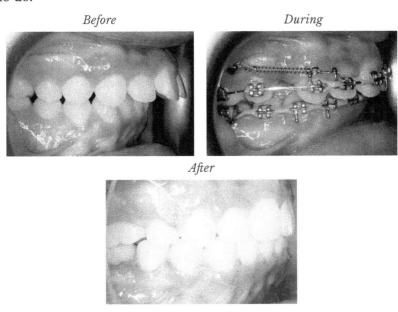

After

Patient presented to us with an excessive overjet and proclined maxillary incisors. Treatment plan included extractions of maxillary first premolars, followed by incisor retraction directly to a TAD.

Like the Herbst, the only extra care needed with a TAD is the same as with braces, watching what you eat and keeping the appliance clean with regular brushing.

SKELETAL PLATES

Skeletal plates, which are placed by an oral surgeon in a minimally invasive procedure, are actually a larger type of TAD. They can be used to apply a force not only to the teeth, but also to the skeletal components. Skeletal plates are sometimes used in conjunction with the smaller TADs.

Before

During

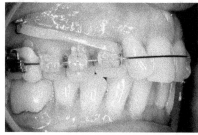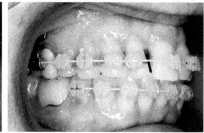

An example of a skeletal plate—for this case, an elastic was worn to the skeletal plate to distalize the posterior teeth into a class I occlusion and provide space to unravel incisor crowding.

BANDS AROUND THE TEETH

In the past, braces often included metal bands that wrapped all the way around each back tooth because it was difficult to get a good bond on the teeth in the back of the mouth. Applying the bands often meant creating space between the teeth with a spacer, a small rubber band that was inserted between the teeth for a few days before being removed ahead of the bands being applied. Now, instead of those bands, we have better technologies that allow for brackets to be bonded, even on the back teeth. Only limited types of appliances, such as those that help break habits, also use bands as part of the system.

ORAL SCANNERS

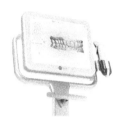 With our oral scanner, we have virtually eliminated the gooey process of making impressions of the teeth. The oral scanner uses a wand to take digital images of the teeth and mouth, which keeps us from having to fill most patients' mouth with gunk. Those digital images allow us to create a virtual 3-D model of the teeth and mouth. The 3-D model gives us an edge when diagnosing and treating patients—we can manipulate the image on the computer to see exactly how the teeth come together and how they can be moved. We can even show the patient a good representation of how their teeth may look at the end of treatment. The model is also used to create appliances and retainers.

NICKEL-TITANIUM WIRES

The wires that we use today are made of nickel titanium, which uses less force than previously used stainless steel wires. That equates to more efficient movement and less soreness in the mouth.

LASER TREATMENT

Laser treatment can reduce inflammation to help alleviate the pain and swelling of puffy gums. The noninvasive laser can also be used to even out the gum line if they are uneven, or to raise the level of the gum line to decrease the appearance of a gummy smile

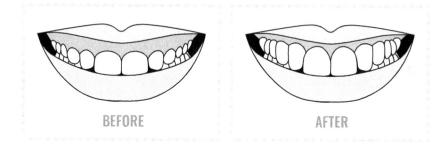

BEFORE   AFTER

CASE STUDY:
SKELETAL PLATE TREATMENT

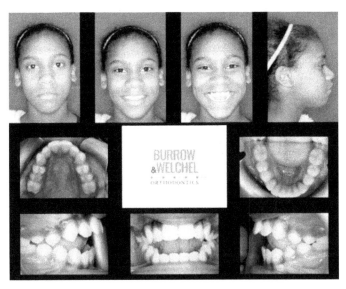

Before: Complex open bite malocclusions were once thought to only to be treated with orthognathic surgery. Today, however, with proper diagnosis and treatment planning, these open bites can be treated predictably with orthodontics alone in growing patients. Proper treatment mechanics are essential to long-term stability and overall esthetics.

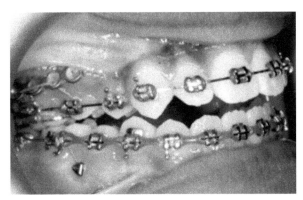

Progress: Posterior intrusion with skeletal plates.

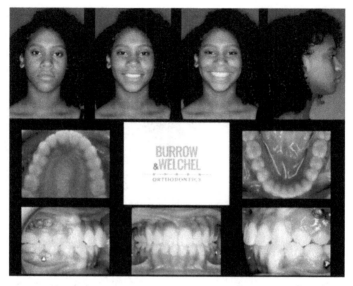

After: This patient's open bite and reverse smile arc were corrected purley through skeletal correction, resulting in a more stable and final occlusion. Posterior intrusion was achieved with skeletal plates and TADs, thus allowing for the mandible to autorotate forward, anterior bite closure, a decrease in lower anterior face height, and a beautiful consonant smile arc.

HOW DO I DEAL WITH "EMERGENCIES"?

Learn when to call the doctor.

WHEN THINGS GO wrong with braces, it can seem like an emergency. And every provider is different in how they handle the problems that arise. Some see patients on weekends, others tell you to wait until Monday to come in. Some have emergency numbers that dial up a treatment coordinator, who usually has you wait until the office opens to be seen. Some charge for emergencies, others don't.

What sets us apart at Burrow & Welchel Orthodontics is that patients are provided with the cell phone number of our doctors and we're happy to meet with you if something is bothering you on the weekend or after hours. Whether we need to clip a wire or repair an appliance, we'll do whatever it takes to make treatment easier on you.

Let's face it: Braces are bonded to the teeth, and as orthodontists, we want the treatment to last as long as we've determined it needs to. But at some point those brackets need to come off, so there is a balancing act when it comes to the bonding—the adhesives have to mimic what we want to happen. So on occasion, eating a hard food or some other activity may cause a bracket to release or a wire to slip out of the bracket and poke the patient in the gums. When that happens, we want patients to know they can reach out to us for help. There's no need to be miserable for days when the problem is usually a very quick fix.

Ideally send a text, or give us a call, and we can set up a time to see you at the office—even after hours.

Here are some emergencies, and some non-emergencies, and what to do about them:

- **An alastic/colored "o-ring" pops off**. These are no big deal—they can wait until the next time the office is open to be seen.

- **A wire is poking you in the gum.** If a wire is poking you in the gum with every bite that you chew, we consider that something that needs to be addressed. Wax applied to the end of the wire or pushing on the wire with a rubber eraser can help, but if those tricks fail to remedy the problem, we want to see you to fix the problem. A rubbing wire can cause a sore spot and, until it's clipped off, can make treatment very uncomfortable.

- **An appliance comes loose and is dangling in the mouth**. This is an emergency that needs to be addressed. This may be the main one we see patients for on weekends.

- **Swelling, abscess, severe pain, or other major discomfort**. Any of these warrant an after-hours call to address whatever is causing the issue.

- **Trauma to the mouth**. This is a true emergency that may even require a trip to the emergency room.

Basically, we want to hear about anything that's bothering you—anything that's causing pain, keeping you from eating, or keeping you from taking part in activities. By reaching out and letting us know what's going on, we can decide whether you need to be seen immediately or whether it's something that can wait.

PART IV:

BRACES FOR ADULTS

AM I TOO OLD FOR BRACES?

Braces aren't just for kids anymore.

BRACES AREN'T JUST for kids anymore. We have patients ranging in age from eight to eighty. In fact, approximately one-third of our patients are adults who have come in to see what can be done to address something they're seeing in the mirror every day. Many end up wearing braces or an appliance to treat their issue.

It's becoming more socially acceptable for adults now to have braces, in part because more people are doing it. For many, getting braces is a lifestyle decision. They're financially stable—their mortgage is paid off, the last of their children are out of the house—so they've got a little more discretionary income. They've seen something in the mirror that has nagged them for years—usually crooked teeth or a smile that needs improvement—so they've decided to do something about it. But not only are braces a good option for adults who want better looking teeth, but realigning a bite or correcting other issues in the mouth can make a huge difference in overall health. Straight teeth are easier to clean, which can keep plaque buildup at bay. That can keep other problems from occurring, such as gum disease and recession, bone loss, and even tooth loss.

One of the most difficult parts of adult treatment is just taking that first step. Adults often delay treatment because of preconceived notions of what braces are all about. Many people believe the only options in braces are the silver metal brackets and wires. They may have worn those as a child and remember the whole experience as very painful, and maybe a little embarrassing. The technologies at that time made the experience less than ideal for many people. But orthodontics has changed over the years.

The visits are more comfortable as well. We start with an initial exam that takes more of a consultative approach. We want to know the chief complaint: What issues do you want addressed? All of these are taken into consideration when putting together a treatment plan. To help with the final decision on treatment, we share the advantages and disadvantages of each option based on your individual situation.

For instance, adults often want to close a gap that has developed in their upper front teeth or to address crowding that has occurred with their lower front teeth. For those who wore braces in the past, the issues are not always severe, so they don't always require two or more years in braces. Sometimes we can correct small issues with braces worn for the short term or with a series of clear aligners.

In that initial consult, we gather all of the records necessary for a thorough diagnosis, including taking a digital scan of the teeth to create a model of the mouth. That's one of the innovations that make treatment a much better experience these days—we no longer fill your mouth with goop to get an impression of your teeth. With the digital scanner, we can create a virtual model that we can even use to predict the outcomes of treatment—we can show you on the computer screen what your teeth will look like at the end of treatment.

Other technologies today that are more appealing to adults include:

- **Nickel-titanium wires**. Today we start treatment with wires made of nickel titanium. They move teeth with continuous, lighter force. That lighter force makes treatment less painful, a real plus for many adults. Then we finish treatment with stainless steel wires, which apply a heavier force.

  The technologies and techniques we use today for moving teeth also mean fewer visits for adjustments than what were required in the past. Treatment timeline is one of the primary concerns of adults, but today's technologies allow us to give many of them the results they're after in less than a year.

- **Clear brackets and wires**. Ceramic braces made of translucent material are a popular choice for adults today. Unlike the older versions of cosmetic brackets, which yellowed over time, the new brackets and wires don't stain easily. They are far less noticeable on teeth.

- **Smaller brackets**. Today's brackets have a lower profile. They are thinner, so they don't stand out from the teeth as far and don't feel as bulky inside the mouth.

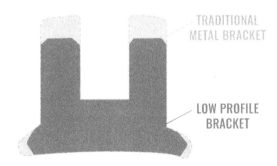

TRADITIONAL METAL BRACKET

LOW PROFILE BRACKET

- **Invisalign**. Invisalign is a brand of clear aligners, or clear plastic "trays," that are customized to the teeth. To straighten teeth, patients are given a series of these aligners. They swap out an aligner each week, and over time, the aligner system gradually shifts teeth into the desired position. The aligners are nearly invisible— that's good news for adults who don't want others to know they're undergoing treatment. The aligners are also removable, so they can be taken out for eating and cleaning. That means there's no need to avoid crunchy or sticky foods or worry about the extra time and effort it takes to keep teeth clean. Advances in Invisalign in recent years also allow for more control over the treatment, which means the treatment can be finished faster and with better accuracy. The results are usually the same as bracket-and-wire braces.

- **Lingual braces**. For adults who want truly invisible treatment, we offer braces that are bonded to the back of the teeth.

- **Finishing touches**. Adult teeth tend to show more wear and tear than youthful teeth. To return some of that youthfulness, we also offer finishing touches known as enameloplasty or contouring. Each tooth has essentially a mirror-image on the other side of the mouth, and contouring can help return the symmetry to the teeth. At the end of treatment for adults, we polish the surfaces and shape the edges of teeth to give the smile an aesthetic, more youthful appearance.

One final benefit of seeking treatment as an adult is that there tends to be more discipline when it comes to retention. Adults tend to be better at following retention protocols to keep their smile and protect their investment.

IS IT TIME TO SEE AN ORTHODONTIST?

Learn some of the reasons adults seek treatment.

ADULTS OFTEN STRUGGLE FOR years with less-than-attractive teeth.

Most of the adults we see had comprehensive treatment as a young adult. Back then, usually twenty or thirty years prior, retention wasn't recommended as often as it is now. It used to be recommended to only wear the retainer for a few years after braces, because it was believed that the teeth stabilized and didn't shift much after that. Now we know that teeth are continually changing. Just like everything else in the body—hair, eyes, skin—teeth are constantly changing. Even if the teeth came in perfectly and did not require corrections with braces as a youth, they still have a tendency to move with age.

Teeth even shift after braces are worn. That's why retention for a lifetime is so crucial to maintaining a smile after braces. Without retention, teeth tend to shift. Sometimes only slightly—a front tooth turns a bit. But in the mirror, to an adult, that one crooked tooth is just adding to their aging appearance.

Some adults seek treatment because they always wanted it but never had the means. Something or someone else always came first—the mortgage, the kids' schooling, or other daily needs. Now that they're financially stable, and maybe even an empty nester, they can afford to do something about their smile.

We also see adults whose dentist recommended treatment for health reasons or before they perform restorative work. It's important that orthodontic tooth movement be completed *before* restorative work (i.e., implants, crowns, or bridges) to ensure the occlusion, or bite, is first finalized. For instance, in the case of a missing tooth that will be replaced with an implant, braces and sometimes auxiliary treatments are needed to create the proper amount of space for the implant to be placed. Orthodontists will ensure that tooth roots are in the best position before an implant is placed, since the roots of teeth on either side of a missing tooth can sometimes tip, causing the roots to also lean into the space where the implant needs to go. Orthodontic treatment can upright the teeth and get the roots into the correct position, out from where the implant needs to be set.

COMPREHENSIVE (OR FULL) TREATMENT

Comprehensive treatment, or full treatment, focuses not only on the alignment of the teeth but also on the function of the bite. In adults seeking comprehensive treatment, the upper and lower teeth are moved into more ideal positions for health, stability, and aesthetics. Comprehensive treatment in adolescents is undergone when all the adult teeth have erupted. In girls, that typically occurs around age eleven, in boys around age twelve.

Comprehensive treatment looks first at how the upper and lower jaws relate to each other. The jaws set the parameters for moving teeth; the jaws can only be changed within certain limits, which are restricted by biology. Using radiographic measurements (X-rays) to determine where corrections need to be made, we can determine whether the movements that the teeth need are within the parameters set by the jaws. If not, we need to look at repositioning the jaws. In growing patients, that repositioning can sometimes be done with appliances. For instance, temporary anchorage devices (TADs) can be used to move a jaw forward or hold a jaw back without having to resort to surgery.

If the movements needed are outside the parameters set by the jaws, orthognathic surgery may be the only way to get the teeth and jaws in the right place.

Here are some of the issues that comprehensive treatment includes:

SPACING

When spacing is the issue, we often look at using anchorage to correct the problem. With anchorage, we attach appliances to existing structures in the mouth and then apply forces to move teeth in precise ways.

Often, correcting a space issue is not just about closing up a gap. For example, we might need to use anchorage to move the lower molars forward while moving the upper front teeth back. We do that to align the teeth top and bottom to correct the bite, not just close a gap between teeth.

Spacing is also about creating the ideal amount of room for the teeth. Each tooth has an ideal width. If a tooth is narrower than it should be, we can use orthodontics to create the ideal space for the tooth and then build up the tooth to the ideal size. As mentioned, we also create ideal space as part of restorative treatment being done by a dentist.

OVERBITE

Overbite describes upper front teeth overlapping the lower front teeth. The ideal overlap is around 25–30 percent. When the upper front teeth completely overlap the lower teeth, the lower teeth can strike the back of the upper teeth when biting down with excessive force, which can damage the lower teeth over time. An overbite can be caused by over-eruption of the lower front teeth, the upper front teeth, or a combination of both (usually a combination is the problem).

OVERJET

Overjet is often mistaken as an overbite. Overjet is when the upper jaw is positioned forward of the lower jaw. It can be caused by a forward upper jaw, a lower jaw positioned too far back, or a combination of both. In adolescents, a Herbst appliance along with other functional appliances can help correct an overjet. The appliance attaches to braces on the upper and lower side teeth and resides inside the mouth. In adults, orthognathic surgery may correct an overjet.

CROSSBITE

Crossbite can be corrected in adolescents with a palatal expander. Generally, a crossbite occurs when the upper jaw is a little narrower than the lower jaw, causing the upper teeth to bite just inside the lower teeth—that's the opposite of a normal bite. Widening the palate, or the upper jaw, can be done on children during Phase I or comprehensive (Phase II) treatment. It is done before growth is complete, because there is a seam in the roof of the mouth known as the mid-palatal suture. Around age fifteen, the fibrous substance in the seam begins to fuse and become immovable. Until that happens, the seam can be expanded to widen the roof of the mouth. The seam remains movable until adolescence. In adults, the seam is fused, so the only options for correcting a crossbite are (a) straightening the teeth and keeping the crossbite, (b) using wires on the upper arch to expand dentally, or (c) turning to orthognathic surgery to reopen the suture.

If the crossbite only affects one tooth, we may be able to correct the problem with braces and elastics or other auxiliary appliances.

To determine whether the suture is fused, we use what's known as the cervical vertebral maturation (CVM) method, which gauges the patient's skeletal maturity. CVM involves analyzing the maturational stage of certain vertebrae in the neck to determine if growth is complete. It is also possible to determine this by taking an X-ray of the hand or the palate itself to see whether fusion has occurred.

CROWDING

Comprehensive treatment corrects crowding by moving and aligning the upper and lower teeth to ensure that the bite fits together. Correcting crowding issues also improves the look of teeth for a more aesthetically pleasing smile.

Correcting crowding problems can also take care of health issues, because straight teeth are much easier to clean. Crowded teeth have a lot of nooks and crannies that are difficult to reach with the bristles of a brush or with floss. Teeth that are not adequately cleaned can get a buildup of plaque, which can cause cavities or even gingivitis, which can turn to periodontitis, which can lead to bone loss and even tooth loss.

To determine whether an extraction is needed to address crowding, we use diagnostic records to look at the bones of the upper and lower jaw that hold the teeth. When teeth are aligned orthodontically, crowding can be eliminated either by tooth movement laterally or forwards. If this movement extends beyond the biological limitation of the bone, the root of the tooth can put too much pressure on the bone and cause it to recede. When the bone recedes, the gums follow. That can lead to tooth instability, as well as the potential for the roots of the teeth to be exposed, resulting in sensitivity.

Instead of trying to fit all the teeth into the arch when there clearly is not enough room—which can cause teeth to flare or result in a "buck tooth" look—we may recommend pulling a tooth to allow enough space to move the teeth into place. The teeth most commonly extracted are the premolars. Depending on our facial goals, we are able to modify treatment to either provide a profile change (i.e., in the case of lip strain or lip protrusion where a "softer" profile is desired) or maintain the existing profile if there is balance and harmony.

In orthodontics, we not only have the ability to change the position of the teeth, but also how the soft tissue overlays the teeth. For example, if a patient presents to our office with lip strain (difficulty fully closing their lips around their teeth, causing the muscles around the mouth to strain) or lip protrusion (a full, or forward position of the lips), it may be our goal to retract the teeth, thus decreasing lip strain or protrusion.

CASE STUDY:
CAMOUFLAGING NANCY'S OVERJET

Sometimes an overjet—when the lower jaw is set back from the upper—can be camouflaged by extracting some of the upper teeth, usually along the sides or back of the mouth, and then retracting the upper incisors. When Nancy came in, the angulation of her lower front teeth was fine, so we didn't need to extract any teeth on the lower arch. But she had a very large overjet and upper teeth that were slightly flared.

By extracting two upper premolars, we were able to use the space to pull the upper teeth back to where they met the lower teeth and corrected her bite. That allowed us to avoid jaw surgery.

Another common reason for an extraction is small upper incisors combined with lower crowding. When there is up to ten millimeters of crowding, we can fix five of it with orthodontic treatment, and the other five we can correct by removing a lower incisor tooth. This works very well both aesthetically and functionally. We have cases available to show patients how the treatment works, because so many are very concerned about removing any teeth—no matter the situation. Adults sometimes lose unhealthy teeth along the way, so when they come in for orthodontic treatment and we're recommending an extraction, it can be shocking to be told that a healthy tooth needs to be taken out. With the tooth out, the remaining teeth fit much better into the existing bone, as opposed to being pushed beyond their limitations. It also makes oral hygiene easier to maintain, which keeps the remaining teeth healthier and causes fewer problems in the future.

Before   *After*

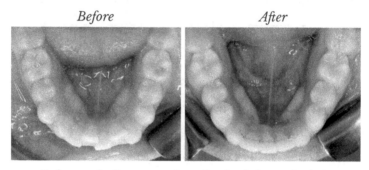

Before and after extraction of a single lower incisor.

Some brackets today advertise that no teeth ever have to be removed. But that's simply not true—no provider can guarantee the best results in all cases without occasionally having to extract teeth. The finished case may look good, but those cases are typically not nearly as stable and can even cause harm if not diagnosed correctly.

Again, the goal is to make a good, healthy bite where the upper and lower teeth all fit together well. That's a stable bite.

WHAT OPTIONS DO YOU HAVE FOR ADULT BRACES?

There are better choices today for adults.

THE PERCENTAGE OF ADULTS wearing braces is going up every year. There is a lot more marketing from some big-name companies raising awareness about the options available, and more people are seeing results in others firsthand and wanting the same for themselves. They're seeing people who once had crooked teeth have renewed smiles and realizing that they never even knew the person had an appliance in their mouth.

Braces are becoming a very popular option for adults looking to regain some youthfulness in their face. Often that's because getting photographed and then having those photos posted online is the norm these days. In fact, in 2017, some 42 percent of facial plastic surgeons reported seeing patients for procedures because they wanted to look better in social media postings.[4]

How does that relate to orthodontics? Many plastic surgery procedures are temporary solutions to age-related changes, compared to the long-term structural changes made with orthodontic procedures.

---

4   "Social Media Continues to Influence Facial Plastic Surgery Requests," news release, June 16, 2017, American Academy of Facial Plastic and Reconstructive Surgery, accessed November 11, 2017, https://www.aafprs.org/media/press-release/20170616.html.

The face changes with aging. Some of those changes are due to the underlying bone structure and tooth position, which affects how the skin and lips appear. Orthodontic treatment can realign teeth and potentially reshape the jaws to create a broader smile and improve the fullness of the lips, giving the face and lips a more youthful look.

Orthodontic treatments also address the wear and tear that is often so visible on adult teeth. By realigning the front teeth and finishing off treatment with contouring or restorative work, we can return the smile line to one that has a more youthful look.

In some adults, another potential impediment to a beautiful smile is excessive gingival display. That's when too much gum tissue shows during a big smile—what's known as a "gummy smile." A gummy smile can be caused by a number of factors, including over-eruption of teeth, excessive vertical movement of the upper jaw during growth, enlarged gum tissues, or any combination of the above. When the teeth are the issue, we can often pull them back into the gums by a few millimeters to recreate a more ideal smile. When there is an excessive vertical growth of the upper jaw, orthognathic surgery may be required to correct the situation. When the issue is enlarged gum tissue, a beautiful result can be obtained by raising the gum line via a procedure known as gingival recontouring, or crown lengthening.

In adults, the distance we can move the teeth to create a broader smile is limited by the width of the bone of the upper jaw. Still, the options we have available create that nice, wide smile and reduce the size of the buccal corridor, those dark spaces that show on either side of the teeth toward the back of the mouth during a smile. Those dark spaces make the smile look narrower—and add to the aging of the face.

Crowded teeth can also add years to a face and potentially create some real oral and overall health problems over time. Yet even when health is a concern, it can be difficult for adults to pursue treatment. That's because adults—and teens—don't want to wear braces that are visible on the teeth.

But take heart: there are some great options today to align teeth, and no one may even realize you're being treated.

CLEAR BRACES VERSUS INVISALIGN

Two of the most popular treatment options for adults include clear ceramic brackets with clear wires and clear aligners such as Invisalign. There are pros and cons to each.

Clear braces are like metal braces in that they use wire to move teeth. That means periodic visits to the orthodontic practice to have the braces adjusted. Like metal braces, they also require more maintenance to keep clean. That means three brushings a day and a daily flossing with a threader or other helper to keep long-term problems from developing. Clear braces are most appropriate for very complex cases and for cases where the patient is too busy (or maybe not disciplined enough) to self-manage the system. Aligners need discipline to be able to wear them the appropriate amount of time per day, or the teeth will not move, whereas braces are fixed and will move the teeth appropriately.

Clear aligners such as Invisalign or 3M Clarity

Aligners can be a great option for aesthetics and for convenience. Clear aligners are easy to maintain because they are removable. Since they are taken out for eating, there are no dietary restrictions.

Treatment with Invisalign is largely self-managed. After a treatment plan is developed by the orthodontist, the trays are created and given to the patient, who switches out the trays weekly over the course of treatment. That means fewer visits to the orthodontist's office during treatment.

Clear aligners are not appropriate for every case. In recent years, however, Invisalign has developed a system that requires small attachments to be placed on teeth, and these have greatly expanded the types of cases that the clear aligners work on, allowing us to treat patients who need more complicated movements. And since the aligners are a self-managed system, they require compliance on the patient's part for the outcome to be successful.

SIX-MONTH BRACES

We also offer a six-month treatment plan using clear brackets and wires. This is only for certain cases, such as adults who didn't wear their braces and had one tooth relapse and get out of alignment. Many relapse cases can be completed in six months. When the treatment won't cause other problems, we will give the patient only what they want—such as realigning that single tooth. If we find another issue during our evaluation, however, we will explain it along with treatment options.

With orthodontics being more efficient today, adult treatment can often be completed in twelve to eighteen months. That's all it takes to get a beautiful smile, one that looks better and is healthier for life.

I HAD BRACES WHEN I WAS YOUNGER, BUT MY TEETH ARE CROOKED AGAIN. WHAT CAN I DO?

*Options today offer easy fixes for relapsed
teeth in some cases.*

A NUMBER OF ADULTS who come in for a consultation are looking for retreatment. They had braces earlier in life but didn't wear their retainers long term, so their teeth have relapsed—they've begun shifting back to their original positions.

Sometimes, however, their relapse has occurred because retention protocol today is different than it was in the past. It used to be believed that once teeth were stabilized with braces, they would stay in position. Now we know that is absolutely not true, because even people who had perfect teeth as a teenager and never wore braces are dealing with shifting teeth as they age.

That happens because the teeth have a tendency to collapse inwards as a person ages and with constant use. That causes the teeth to crowd and begin turning or tilting to accommodate all the changes. Most of the time, the crowding occurs in the lower front teeth.

TEETH MOVE—THAT'S CERTAIN

Teeth crowd and become turned and crooked for a number of reasons. When there isn't enough room in the jawbone for all the teeth, they can crowd while coming in. That happens in children and adolescents.

There are multiple surges in tooth movement—one occurring between ages seventeen and twenty-one at roughly the same time that the wisdom teeth start to come in, when the last of the permanent teeth erupt into the mouth. That makes people want to point to the eruption of wisdom teeth as the reason for teeth moving and growing crooked. But the two events are actually not related. Erupting molars don't necessarily dictate whether teeth will crowd. Teeth can crowd even in patients who are missing their wisdom teeth.

Invisalign Express. In some cases, Invisalign Express is a potential option for a quick, painless retreat of teeth that have relapsed. Invisalign Express involves ten weeks of trays (ten trays, one per week) that move one or two teeth back into the correct position.

The bottom line with teeth is that without treatment they will continue to move. The more they move, the more problems they can cause. And treating crowding sooner typically means treatment takes less time.

WANT STRAIGHT TEETH? WEAR RETAINERS

Just as other parts of the body change over time—your hair changes, your skin changes—teeth are no different. Teeth move with time. But by having orthodontic treatment and then wearing a retainer for life, teeth can stay in position for the long term.

At Burrow & Welchel Orthodontics, we recommend that everyone wear retainers for life. That means that as long as you want to have straight teeth, you need to wear your retainers at night.

Following treatment, we see patients once or twice in the nine months after the braces are removed to ensure that retainers fit and are retaining the position of the teeth. After that, retainers are replaced on an as-needed basis, and if a retainer is lost we recommend getting it replaced as soon as possible. If you lose a retainer, it won't take long before you will notice a difference in the way it fits. Often, it will feel tight after a couple of days without wearing it. If that happens, we usually suggest wearing it full time again for a couple of days, then going back to nighttime protocol. If it feels too loose, you may need to come in and get it checked. If you find at some point that it doesn't go on at all, that means that your teeth have shifted to where you need another retainer or maybe some more treatment.

While some people can wear the same retainer for decades, we recommend at least having retainers checked, if not replaced, at minimum every five years. Think of them like eyeglasses—you wouldn't want to try to see through the same lenses for twenty years, would you?

PART V:

THE BRACES FEAR FACTOR

DO BRACES HURT?

Improved technologies make braces a more comfortable experience.

THE FEAR OF PAIN keeps a lot of people from pursuing braces as a treatment for their orthodontic problems. But technologies have advanced so much over the years that there is far less pain or discomfort than treatments of the past.

For instance, when we start treatment, the wires we use apply a light, continuous force, which results in less pain. When the force on teeth is too strong, as it was with wires in the past, it can block the blood flow to the area and cause what's known as undermining resorption. Basically, that means the site where the tooth is trying to move in the bone gets a buildup of substance that must first be broken down to make room for the tooth. After the body's cells migrate to the area to break down that substance, the tooth moves very quickly—that's what causes pain. When light force is applied, the teeth move steadily, at the right speed, and that undermining resorption process doesn't occur. That's why light forces move teeth faster.

There may still be some pain in some patients after an adjustment, but that pain tends to dissipate in most people after twenty-four hours and should be totally alleviated within about three days.

If rubber bands are part of the treatment plan, but they are only used sporadically instead of being worn daily and switched out twice a day as recommended, the treatment can be more painful. But any discomfort from the bands subsides after a couple of days at most.

Other technologies that reduce the discomfort of orthodontics include a scanner that takes images of the teeth and is used to create the 3-D model of the patient's mouth. This technology means that we no longer have to fill your mouth with goop to make an impression—the old method of creating molds has by itself kept some people from getting treatment in the past.

DEALING WITH PAIN

For patients who tend to be more sensitive to pain, we recommend taking an over-the-counter pain medicine such as Advil or Tylenol an hour before their appointment so that it kicks in when needed.

If there is already a sore or ulcer in the mouth, braces rubbing on the spot can worsen the problem. For these issues, we recommend applying wax, Gishy Goo, or OrthoDots to the bracket or wire that's causing the problem. Gishy Goo is a liquid that hardens after it is molded around the bracket to act like a pillow or cushion to protect the insides of the lips and cheeks. OrthoDots are small dots of silicone that can be applied where needed.

Even with today's lower-profile brackets, there can be some soreness at the beginning of treatment anywhere the brackets rub. Like breaking in a new pair of shoes, if a blister forms but you continue to wear the shoes, the blister will heal and no longer be painful. With time, your mouth adapts and you won't get those ulcers as frequently or at all.

Other remedies include Orajel to help to numb the area and medicated rinses like Peroxyl, which we supply as part of our new-patient kits. Even rinsing with warm saltwater will help to cleanse the area and ensure faster healing.

DO YOUR PART

Keeping your teeth clean and gums healthy during treatment can also help reduce pain. Gums should not bleed; if they do, it means there is infection present. Complications during treatment such as gingivitis or gum infections can make treatment more painful.

Lack of good oral hygiene can even impede tooth movement in extreme cases. For instance, plaque left on the teeth can turn to calculus, which can actually act like a concrete bridge between teeth and prevent their movement.

Having orthodontic treatment today is a much more comfortable experience overall than in the past. And as orthodontists, we're very conscious of our patients' comfort and do what we can to make the process as enjoyable as possible.

WILL I NEED TO HAVE TEETH PULLED?

Maybe. Read why, and why not.

THE BEST ANSWER? Maybe.

There is a lot of misinformation about this topic. Many people believe that crowding or aesthetic desires often lead to having teeth extracted. While those issues can involve extractions, that's not always the case. There are more options today to help us move teeth and bone in ways that allow us to keep the teeth intact.

A note of caution: There are claims that some types of brackets never require having teeth extracted. That is simply not the case. There are no brackets on the market for which it can be guaranteed that teeth will never need to be extracted.

Case in point: Self-ligating brackets are a type of bracket that has a "gate" that closes down over the wire to hold it in place throughout treatment. There are claims that self-ligating brackets allow for greater widening of the arch of the jaw to allow more teeth to remain in place instead of having to extract them to alleviate crowding. There are also claims that since the gate means no rubber bands are required to hold the wire in place, there is less friction when moving teeth and therefore less pain. For instance, the Damon system is one example of a self-ligating bracket and is notorious for claiming that, if this bracket system is used, it will decrease the need for extractions because it allows for "arch development" a.k.a. expansion. However, expansion is not always a good thing! Excessive expansion may push a tooth beyond the confines of its bony housing, causing perforations in the bone and gum recession.

But teeth don't know the difference between self-ligating brackets and twin brackets. Twin brackets are the style of bracket that has "wings" that rubber bands attach onto. Those bands hold the wire in place on each bracket.

The truth is that teeth move at the same rate with twin brackets as with self-ligating brackets, and there is the same amount of discomfort with either. And no system allows for the jaw arch to be widened beyond safe and stable biological limits.

When it comes to extractions at Burrow & Welchel Orthodontics, we take a conservative approach. We want to avoid extractions if at all possible, but sometimes they are absolutely necessary to provide the most aesthetic smile and the most functional bite.

To determine whether extractions are needed, we look at issues such as the angulation of the teeth. Do teeth need to be removed to prevent them from protruding or flaring? Can we achieve the optimum angles on the teeth without taking any others out? We also look at the health of the gum tissue and underlying bone. By considering all these factors, we can create a treatment plan to keep the teeth and mouth stable and healthy for the long term.

In some cases, extractions are needed to keep from pushing teeth beyond their biological limits and overexpanding the arch or causing the teeth to tilt outward. When that happens, teeth are more inclined to try to move back to their initial position, making the bite less stable and less healthy.

Before *After*

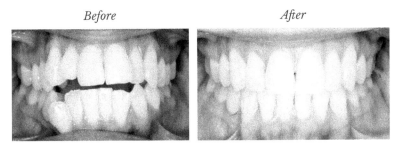

Before and after extractions to resolve crowding and correct an open bite.

CASE STUDY:
CLOSING SANDRA'S OPEN BITE

Sandra was in her early twenties when she came in with a slight open bite—a gap between her upper and lower front teeth when she closed her mouth. She already had very full lips, so our goal was a treatment plan designed to reduce the lip protrusion by retracting her teeth slightly. That would allow for a balanced profile and eliminate lip strain upon closure. The treatment would also help close her open bite. By extracting some teeth, we were able to retract the remaining teeth, moving them back to close the gap in her bite and upright her teeth. That also allowed her lips to relax and close easily over her teeth.

CASE STUDY:
ALLEVIATING LORI'S SEVERE CROWDING

When Lori's mother brought her in for treatment, the young girl already had severe upper and lower crowding of her teeth. In her case, it made sense to extract some teeth and redistribute the remaining teeth to prevent her front teeth from flaring. We extracted four premolars, one on each side of the upper and lower arches of her jaws. Then we used the space to move Lori's canines back. That allowed us to unravel the crowding in the other front teeth, letting them line up into a beautiful smile.

HOW WE SEE WHAT'S GOING ON

Today's technologies help us determine when extractions are required.

We take full records on every patient, including one that is known as a lateral cephalometric radiograph or X-ray. From that X-ray, we're able to perform an analysis that shows us the angles of the teeth related to each jaw, to each other, and to the skull. The X-ray also shows how the jaws relate to each other.

The "ceph," as it is often called, also allows us to set up a digital, virtual plan to simulate where the teeth will move. Then we can determine which teeth need to come out and what space is available to redistribute the remaining teeth.

WILL I NEED TO HAVE JAW SURGERY?

It depends on your case.

THERE IS A lot of misinformation out there about jaw surgery. Some providers of orthodontic treatment claim to be able to move teeth and jaws without ever needing jaw surgery.

But there are certain limits to purely orthodontic tooth movement. On average, with orthodontic movement alone we can typically move teeth about six millimeters, just under a quarter inch. If a patient comes in with a very severe overjet, or jaws that don't line up into the ideal bite, we have to determine whether the underlying issue is caused by the teeth, the jaws, or a combination of both. Depending on our findings, we may recommend surgery to correct a structural issue before we align the bite.

Children and teens have growth on their side, so treatments can correct some issues without surgery. This growth can be used to correct jaw discrepancies in three planes of space: the vertical, anterior-posterior (or front to back), and transverse dimensions. For instance, in the case of excessive overjet, a Herbst appliance can be placed to help restrict growth of the upper jaw and accelerate growth of the lower jaw. If the skeletal discrepancy is severe, sometimes it can't be completely corrected with a growth-modification appliance alone. In a case like that, surgery is still required for that last bit of correction. As discussed before, in the case of a crossbite due to constriction of the upper jaw, it is possible in a growing patient to expand the suture that runs down the palate. However, in adults, the suture becomes very complex and is no longer patent, thus prohibiting skeletal expansion with appliances. At that age, surgical intervention is sometimes required for expansion of the palate.

There are numerous benefits of surgical orthodontics. Not only can it improve overall facial aesthetics to create a more balanced profile, it may also be recommended to improve function. For instance, it can correct a gummy smile, where a large amount of gum shows when someone smiles, which can occur when the upper jaw grows further down than normal during development. Surgery can correct a gummy smile by raising the upper jaw. If needed, the jaw can also be widened at the same time. Surgery in adults can also correct front-to-back discrepancies in jaws. For instance, if a patient has an underbite, the entire upper jaw can be moved forward or the lower jaw can be moved backward.

The aesthetic result of widening the jaw is a broader smile, one that fills the buccal corridors. The buccal corridors are those dark areas between the teeth and cheek tissues at the back of the mouth when a person smiles. Filling the dark corridors can create a more youthful smile.

NO TO SURGERY? WE CAN STILL HELP

Some patients have no interest in undergoing jaw surgery. The technologies available today allow us to offer a compromise treatment plan that lines up the teeth but maintains some issues such as an overbite or crossbite that can only be addressed with surgery. These compromise treatments are still an improvement for the patient, one that they understand fully and approve in advance. And they usually leave the door open for surgery in the future, should the patient change their mind.

Compromise treatment is also an option for adults, since they don't have the flexibility of using a palatal expander for correction of a narrow maxillary arch (maxillary arch meaning upper jaw, and mandibular meaning lower jaw). Remember, the mid-palatal suture is fused in adulthood and can only be reopened surgically. However, it is possible to expand teeth to a certain limit to slightly broaden the smile. Beyond those limits, detrimental things can happen to the surrounding bone and gum tissue. An adult with a posterior crossbite who did not have orthodontic treatment as a child may require some sort of surgical intervention for full crossbite correction if the limits of orthodontic tooth movement alone is reached.

HOW MUCH DO BRACES COST?

Treatment determines the cost, you decide the value.

THE COST OF braces depends on the treatment. Basic costs of treatment are approximately the same for both bracket-and-wire braces and clear aligners. One advantage to the clear aligner therapy, such as Invisalign treatment, is that it requires fewer visits to the office. So, if minimizing time in the office is a factor and the treatment plan will support using aligners, that option may be a good choice.

The severity of the case determines the treatment complexity, and that typically determines the cost. For instance, temporary anchorage devices (TADs), skeletal plates, Herbst appliances, and Forsus springs are used for specific, more complex movements. Surgery, longer treatment times, and complications such as an impacted tooth are other kinds of issues that may warrant a higher treatment fee.

What's key to remember when it comes to cost is that even though the technologies have greatly improved, the cost of being in braces has not risen to match the advances. What other medical procedure—or what other area of life—can say the same?

The good news is that everyone doesn't need comprehensive treatment. Sometimes treatment can involve just tweaking some crowding in the lower front teeth or closing up space between the upper front teeth. If that's all that's needed, or if the patient only wants limited treatment and it won't cause other problems, then we do everything we can to help them accomplish their goals. Costs for that limited treatment are significantly less than a full fee.

Since orthodontic treatment takes longer than most dental procedures, most orthodontists offer a complimentary monthly payment plan that lasts the duration of the treatment and can help keep payments low.

WHAT ARE YOUR TEETH WORTH TO YOU?

Orthodontic treatment goes beyond the dollars spent. It is the best investment you can make. It's an investment in good oral health and a good bite, and something that will be with you for the rest of your life.

Straight teeth are easier to keep clean, helping to avoid the buildup of plaque, which can lead to gum disease over time. Research is now looking at the link between gum disease and other diseases of the body including diabetes and heart disease. With both diseases, inflammation is being targeted as the culprit, and with diabetes the connection appears to go both ways—diabetics are more prone to gum disease, and gum disease makes it harder to keep diabetes in check.[5] Studies have also found a link between gum disease and other issues such as respiratory problems and even cancer.[6]

Beyond the health issue, studies have found that orthodontics can also enhance self-esteem and improve a person's social life. People with a severely malaligned bite tend to have more trouble with social interactions and are more likely to be teased. But their problems tend to improve once they have orthodontic treatment, largely due to their improved smile.[7]

---

5   "Diabetes and Periodontal Disease," American Academy of Periodontology, accessed April 10, 2018, https://www.perio.org/consumer/gum-disease-and-diabetes.htm.

6   "Gum Disease and Other Systemic Diseases," American Academy of Periodontology, accessed April 10, 2018, https://www.perio.org/consumer/other-systemic-diseases.

7   John Roger Feusier, "Does orthodontic treatment in adolescents affect quality of life? A practice-based research model."

In a study commissioned by Invisalign, nearly a third of participants (29 percent) said that teeth were the first thing they noticed about a person, and nearly a quarter (24 percent) said teeth were the feature they remembered most about a person.[8] Participants in the study were shown images of people and asked to give their opinions about them. The people in the images had various issues with their teeth—some were straight, some were not. But participants in the study were not told that they were judging people based on their smile. Most of the respondents (73 percent) said they thought a person with a nice smile was more trustworthy, and some 38 percent said they thought people with nice smiles were smarter. Nearly half (45 percent) thought that the person with straight teeth would be more likely to be offered a job over a person with crooked teeth. And more than half (58 percent) were perceived as being wealthier and more successful.[9] In another survey of singles and relationships, men and women placed the appearance of a person's teeth at the top of the list when it came to choosing a potential date.[10]

As the body ages, the soft tissues of the face change. The lips become thinner, and the nose and chin become more prominent. That gives the illusion that a person is losing volume in their lips—which makes them look older. As that volume decreases, it also conceals the gum tissues, which can add to an aging face. By placing the teeth in a position that provides a foundation for the lips, their volume can be

8   "First Impressions Are Everything: New Study Confirms People with Straight Teeth Are Perceived as More Successful, Smarter and Having More Dates," PR Newswire, Apr 19, 2012, accessed March 2, 2018, https://www.prnewswire.com/news-releases/first-impressions-are-everything-new-study-confirms-people-with-straight-teeth-are-perceived-as-more-successful-smarter-and-having-more-dates-148-073735.html.

9   Ibid.

10   Jayson, Sharon, "What singles want: Survey looks at attraction, turnoffs," USA Today, February 5, 2013, accessed January 11, 2018, https://www.usatoday.com/story/news/nation/2013/02/04/singles-dating-attraction-facebook/1878265.

maintained long term. People pay tens of thousands of dollars every year on plastic surgery to improve their looks. But plastic surgery is often temporary, whereas orthodontic treatment followed by a retention program can give you a youthful smile forever.

HOW DO I PAY FOR BRACES?

Insurance for some, financing options for others.

AT BURROW & WELCHEL Orthodontics, our treatment coordinators discuss all the financial aspects of treatment to help you understand your options and give you choices that work with your budget.

We are in-network with a number of insurance companies, which helps to lower the overall cost of treatment and make it more affordable. Not all insurance policies include orthodontic coverage, and some have a one-year waiting period—those details are checked before treatment begins.

For patients who self-pay, we offer zero percent financing over the course of treatment, and it's all done in-house. We allow you to make payments throughout the course of treatment, which is a big plus for many families. The payments are less than a cell phone bill and can be determined by the amount of down payment made at the beginning of treatment. For example, a larger payment at the start of treatment can make monthly payments even more affordable. We also offer a discount for paying in full on the day the braces are placed.

The fees for treatment are all-inclusive. The cost determined up front includes all of the visits, all of the treatments, and observation to check retention at three and six months after treatment.

PART VI:

BRACES—THE EXPERIENCE

WHAT CAN I EXPECT AT MY INITIAL EXAM?

What it's like to be a patient at
Burrow & Welchel Orthodontics.

AT THE INITIAL EXAM, you are greeted by our friendly front desk staff. Staff members welcome you to the office, check you in, and make sure all your new patient paperwork is filled out. That paperwork includes medical history, insurance information, and other details we'd like to know before beginning the consult. New patient paperwork is typically mailed and emailed before the first exam to allow time to fill it out in advance so the process is more seamless.

Then a treatment coordinator greets you and acts as your tour guide for the day. The coordinator gives you an overview of the practice, talks with you about the doctors, and tells you what to expect when meeting with the doctors. The coordinator will gather diagnostic information including digital photos, X-rays, digital models (sometimes), and any other records that may be needed for formulation of a thorough treatment plan.

One or more of our doctors then comes in to meet with you, perform a clinical exam, and evaluate the records that were taken. The doctor or doctors go over any issues that are found. Most of the time, the doctors can formulate a diagnosis at that time.

The doctor then leaves the room and lets the treatment coordinator discuss the different types of braces and some of the pros and cons of the treatment options.

The entire visit is complimentary, no fees. It's not very often that you are able to be seen by a medical professional for an initial diagnosis and opinion free of charge.

For those cases that are fairly straightforward, we may even begin treatment that same day—a welcome convenience for many patients.

When a case is more complex, treatment may begin on a second visit to the office, during which the consult involves a formal discussion of treatment options. What sets Burrow & Welchel apart is that between the two visits, all three doctors in our practice come together to create a customized plan, since no two mouths are alike. Our team approach integrates the expertise of all three highly trained orthodontists into individual treatment plans.

Treatment takes place in one of seven semiprivate bays. Each bay is divided by a partition that helps retain privacy but adds to the energy of the practice, since we're all in one room together.

Our offices are fun, positive, and very upbeat. Since patients are seen roughly every eight weeks, we like to try to match chair-side assistants with patients to improve continuity during treatment. That also allows us to build better relationships with patients, to get to know each patient as an individual.

In fact, our goal is to help you get comfortable with our office, our staff, and the overall family atmosphere that you'll find here. We want to get to know you and help you feel secure in your choice of orthodontists, because we're going to be together for quite some time. The average length of time for non-extraction cases is typically eighteen to twenty-four months and those that require an extraction can take anywhere from twenty-four to thirty-six months. Everyone's case is different, depending on the severity of any malalignment with their teeth and bite.

That's especially helpful for teens, since it's such an important time in their lives. Many patients are receiving treatment during the sixth to ninth grade, and we get to see them transform from a timid middle schooler with less-than-ideal teeth to a high schooler with a bright, confident smile. It's really wonderful to witness.

HOW CAN YOU TELL WHERE
TO MOVE MY TEETH?

3-D imaging lets us better diagnose and treat patients.

DIAGNOSTICS TODAY ALLOW for a better picture of what is going on in the jaw, which helps us be more predictive with treatment.

By looking at the results of diagnostic testing—including digital photography of the teeth and face, 3-D images of the jaws, and a hundred years of research of similar cases—we can see any complications under the gum line that could affect treatment. We can also see complications that might cause the teeth to relapse after treatment without retention.

The 3-D technologies that we use today also allow us to move the teeth virtually to create the best treatment plan. Getting that virtual picture of movement results in healthier outcomes in part because the teeth are moved more efficiently—we're able to predict when moving one tooth may cause other teeth to move. With adolescents and adults, we can also predict stability norms. In other words, we can look at where the patient's teeth started before movement began.

By getting a better picture of what's going on in the mouth, we're able to move the teeth in a predictable way to help with aesthetics, stability, and maintaining the health of the teeth and bite.

The 3-D imaging lets us see all planes of space. We can see everything from the root to the crown and exactly how teeth are angulated in the mouth. In the case of problems like impactions, we can now see the tooth beneath the gum tissue and in the bone—that gives us a much better understanding of how to move the tooth into the mouth in a healthy, more efficient manner that won't harm other teeth. In the past, since 2-D images did not always let us see the exact location of all the teeth concealed under the gum line, treatment efficiency was not always maximized when moving an impacted tooth into place. But now we can make impacted movements much quicker and more predictably, because we can apply the proper force and force vector.

The cone beam computed tomography (CBCT) images hard tissue from the neck up, allowing us to see the jaws and entire skull in three dimensions. The scan takes only a few seconds and then gives us a virtual image of the teeth that we can turn in every direction on the computer screen, ensuring a complete diagnosis is determined. Also, using 3-D software on the digital scanner, we can also virtually move the teeth into place before beginning treatment. With a few clicks, we can virtually straighten all the teeth and, during the consultation, predict what the teeth will look like when they are all lined up. It's a great tool for treatment planning and fun for patients to see. It's pretty exciting when they can see their crowded teeth aligned into a beautiful smile. It's a little like using an app to try out a new hairstyle before getting a cut and color.

A lot of people don't even know the extent of their mal-aligned bite until they see it on the screen. Then showing them how their teeth are expected to move during treatment reassures them that the treatment plan is on track and lets them visualize how much movement needs to occur for their teeth to be straightened out.

WILL I TALK FUNNY IN BRACES?

After a couple of days, you'll adjust.

A LOT OF PEOPLE, especially adult patients, are concerned about the potential impact of braces on their ability to speak, since they have to talk a lot on the phone, at their job, or in a professional setting. The truth is, you will sound worse to yourself than you do to others, because everyone is their own worst critic.

When the braces are first placed on the teeth, it can take a day or two to get accustomed to them. If you feel uncomfortable speaking, we recommend going home and reading a favorite book out loud for fifteen minutes. That allows your body to adapt to wearing the fixed braces or clear aligner appliance.

After a couple of days, it's pretty easy to adjust to braces or aligners and they become a part of your everyday life.

HOW WILL BRACES AFFECT MY LIFESTYLE?

Invisible, yes, but they still need extra care.

TECHNOLOGIES ARE SO much better today that they make having braces a far less intrusive experience overall. Options are designed to be practically invisible, and include:

Ceramic brackets and wires. These work just like metal brackets and wires, but they are nearly invisible and don't stain easily. People often don't even realize that a patient is wearing this option. Ceramic braces are also less bulky than in the past, which makes them more comfortable inside the mouth, so they feel less "clumsy" when eating and speaking.

Invisalign is a brand of clear aligners that are removable for eating and cleaning. These are worn twenty-one hours a day but are custom fitted to the teeth and made of clear plastic, so they are practically invisible.

Lingual brackets are invisible from the front, because they are bonded to the back of the teeth. These can be a little more difficult to get accustomed to, so they may not be the best option for patients who talk for a living—such as people in customer service or sales positions. But they're very appealing to patients in professions where appearances are crucial, such as actors or television personalities.

Auxiliary appliances today are also far less intrusive. Many are attached inside the mouth—instead of being visible on the outside, like headgear—and they make movements of teeth far more precise. These include the Herbst appliance, skeletal plates, Forsus springs, and temporary anchorage devices (TADs). These appliances eliminate concerns over patient compliance, but like braces, they require extra care.

CARE MEASURES

Once you are in braces, they do require more attention to oral hygiene regimen.

Before putting you in an appliance, we stipulate that you must continue regular visits to the dentist during treatment. When you come in for a visit, we pay particular attention to your oral hygiene—we want to see that you are brushing regularly and have no active gingivitis, periodontitis, bone disease, or other issues.

When you have an appliance in your mouth, there is greater surface area for food to get stuck in, and plaque to build up on. Whether you are in brackets and wires or in aligners, we recommend brushing three times a day—after meals and before bedtime. We also recommend flossing once per day. With brackets and wires, flossing is typically done at night, because it takes a bit longer to floss around the brackets and wires. Brushing and flossing with aligners is easier, of course, since the trays themselves are removable.

With either braces or aligners, you may find yourself toting around a brush and floss to care for your teeth after a meal. Teeth move more efficiently in a clean environment—in a clean mouth, biological factors can work a lot better to move the teeth.

When it comes to food, aligners win out over braces. Since aligners are removed for eating, there are no special dietary restrictions. However, it's a good idea with aligners to have a case with you at all times to hold the appliance when it's removed—this can keep it from getting lost or tossed out with the table napkins.

Braces, however, do come with food restrictions. Sticky foods should be avoided, and crunchy foods should be eaten with care. Raw carrots and apples, for instance, should be cut into bite-size pieces. The key is to be mindful of any excess pressure being applied to the bracket—which can cause the bracket to break.

We also recommend avoiding popcorn altogether with braces, since the husks can get caught in inconvenient places and lead to plaque buildup. Other items to avoid include ice and hard candies.

SMALL PRICE FOR A BIG SMILE

Once you have your teeth aligned, we recommend "nighttime for a lifetime" in terms of retention. After treatment is complete, you will have a great, winning smile—in that regard, your life is very much changed. Keeping that smile means wearing retainers every night and replacing them periodically.

If you have a mouthful of malaligned teeth that are making you unhappy and unhealthy, having braces for a relatively short time is a small intrusion for long-term results.

CAN I PLAY SPORTS WHILE WEARING BRACES?

How to protect your teeth during play.

WHERE WE PRACTICE, we get this question a lot. There are a lot of youth sports teams, especially basketball, football, and now lacrosse, all of which are known as high-impact sports. But the list doesn't stop there: baseball, soccer, and other sports also come with the risk of being bumped in the mouth. When that happens, it can be quite painful, but a lot of damage can also happen. Besides the frustration of having to fit in another visit to the orthodontist for a repair, damaged braces can potentially delay treatment.

Braces actually protect the teeth during play. It's easier for a single tooth to be knocked out during play if it is not being held to other teeth with brackets and wires. But where the pain and damage often occur is to the soft tissues of the mouth—the insides of the lip and cheek.

For anyone involved in team sports, we recommend wearing a mouth guard customized for use with braces to protect the teeth and soft tissues of the mouth.

These are not the boil-and-bite mouth guards found at sporting goods stores. Those tend to adhere to the braces, and when removed, they have a tendency to pull the braces off. The mouth guards we recommend are designed to protect the braces and teeth while also providing a protective layer between the teeth and the soft tissues.

PART VII:

LIFE AFTER BRACES

DO I HAVE TO WEAR RETAINERS?

Only if you want straight teeth!

THERE'S AN OLD JOKE in the orthodontics world about wearing retainers: The patient asks the doctor, "How long do I have to wear a retainer?" to which the doctor replies, "How long do you want straight teeth?"

The fact is that teeth move, so retention is key to keeping a great smile at the end of treatment. Retainers protect the investment in braces. In fact, the retention portion of treatment is, on some levels, another diagnosis, because keeping the teeth in the same place as they were at the end of treatment is such a big part of the outcome. We don't just straighten your teeth and send you on your way. We give you an individualized custom retention plan that includes nine months of follow-up after treatment. We make you part of the orthodontic family and encourage you to reach out if there are any issues that need to be addressed.

Retention is so critical to long-term success that the retainer discussion is held at the onset of treatment. We discuss retainers in the appointment when the braces are placed on the teeth, then we continue to reiterate their importance throughout treatment. That way, when the braces are removed, there are no surprises about the fact that retainers must be worn to keep the beautiful smile that braces achieved.

While some orthodontic offices have one retention protocol that is used on every patient, we have several different protocols that tailor retention to the patient's specific needs. Which protocol is used depends on factors such as the original diagnosis, whether the teeth have a higher potential for relapse, and which protocol is likely to be most comfortable and easiest for the patient to use. Again, without retainers, teeth will move, so the decision regarding which protocol to use is based partly on compliance, but is mostly customized to ensure the least relapse potential.

Most patients receive their retainers one week after braces are removed. Patients who have a high relapse potential, however, receive retainers the same day their braces are removed.

When the retainers are delivered to the patient, we ensure that they fit properly and provide instructions on how to keep them clean. We want the patient to understand how to care for them so that they last as long as possible.

There are different opinions about how long retainers must be worn. Some orthodontists believe that wearing a retainer only a couple of nights a week is enough to hold teeth in place once the movements are complete.

Whether a teen or an adult, we share this message about retainers: It takes a lot of time, effort, and expense to move teeth into the right positions. Moving a tooth into a position that it wasn't in before is going against nature to some degree. Since it was moved from one place to another, there is the very real chance that it will want to move back. That's why we need a commitment to retention protocol before treatment even begins. Retention, in essence, is part of treatment— it's part of the lifestyle of having teeth moved. Without retention, the teeth may only move back a little, but the likelihood that they will move is great. That's why we propose wearing retainers "nighttime for a lifetime."

Typically, patients wear retainers full time following treatment. At the three-month point, we check the stability of the teeth and reduce nearly everyone to nighttime-only retention. The first year after braces are removed is the most critical when it comes to retention. During that year, the soft and hard tissues surrounding the teeth are reorganizing and stabilizing. Until that first year is complete, teeth are especially susceptible to relapse.

Over time, retainers tend to wear out or get lost and need to be replaced. If you've ever worn eyeglasses, you understand the concept of replacing a needed aid. Once a person begins wearing eyeglasses, they'll wear them every day to be able to see but will take them off at night. Similarly, after the initial period, orthodontic patients won't wear their retainer during the day, but they are responsible for wearing their retainer at night to keep their teeth straight. And just like glasses, which must be renewed over time, retainers need to be changed out over time.

At our practice, retainers are included in the treatment fee. If a patient of record—someone we've treated—loses a retainer, then only a lab fee is charged. The fees for the doctor and material are waived. That's how much we want patients to keep their teeth straight. The discount is significant compared to the cost for a patient who comes to us only for a retainer.

WHAT IF I DON'T FOLLOW THE DOCTOR'S ORDERS AFTER TREATMENT?

Without retention, your teeth will move.

ONCE THE BRACES are off, patients are ecstatic to see their beautiful smile and get on with their life with sparkling, straight teeth and a healthy, aligned bite. But the treatment doesn't stop once the braces are removed. Without wearing retainers as prescribed by the orthodontist, teeth can relapse or attempt to move back to the position they were in before treatment.

Most relapse occurs in patients who had braces before but didn't wear their retainers. One reason that teeth move is that the gingival fibers that surround teeth rearrange during treatment. Some of those fibrous tissues rearrange better than others, and those that don't will try to pull the tooth back to its original position. It's those few stubborn ligaments that require retention to keep the teeth from moving back, which can lead to crowding or turning and tilting of the teeth.

Just like other areas of the body—hair and skin, for instance—teeth can change position over time. When teeth have been overexpanded beyond their biological limits (i.e., with the Damon philosophy), the arch has the potential to collapse back to its original form.

But teeth move even if braces were never worn. Today we see adults who had perfectly straight teeth in their youth and never wore braces, but now they're coming in to have crooked teeth straightened. That's because the bones and tissues in the body are always reorganizing, which keeps the teeth in constant motion.

When there is crowding in the mouth, typically the lower front teeth are affected the most. To help patients visualize the critical nature of adhering to retention protocol, we sometimes show them photos of teeth that shifted after only six months without wearing a retainer. It can have a great impact on patients to see that kind of change in teeth over such a short period of time, especially for someone who has just had their braces removed.

Should a retainer be lost, it's important to obtain a replacement. Dramatic shifts in the teeth can occur even within a few days after losing a retainer, especially if braces were recently removed. But waiting too long can be detrimental—a week's wait can easily turn into months, and then years. And the longer the time without a retainer, the more shifting that may occur, and the more treatment, time, and expense that may be needed to move the teeth back again.

At Burrow & Welchel Orthodontics, we offer various configurations of retainers, customized to each individual patient. Whichever retainers are used, we recommend that patients wear them every night for the rest of their lives—nighttime for a lifetime, we call it.

PART VIII:

CHOOSING A PROVIDER

HOW DO I FIND THE BEST ORTHODONTIST FOR MY NEEDS?

Here are some tips to use in your search for a provider.

WE KNOW THAT you have choices when it comes to orthodontic providers. To ensure that you're getting someone who understands your specific needs and can provide you a customized solution, we've listed some points to consider when looking for an orthodontist:

Board Certification. Credentials matter when it comes to orthodontists—all orthodontists are not created equal. There are various levels of training, but those orthodontists who hold themselves to a higher standard of orthodontic care have earned board certification. Board certification requires the orthodontist to undergo a rigorous program of demonstrating to peers that they have the knowledge and expertise to deliver superior patient care. Certification must be renewed every ten years.

Orthodontist vs. General Dentist. When it comes to orthodontic treatment, choose someone who moves teeth (an orthodontist) all day long over someone for whom moving teeth is a sideline.

General dentists are trained to manage the health of teeth—to do fillings, crowns, dentures, and more. Orthodontists, on the other hand, are trained specifically in the complex biology involved in moving teeth.

Relatable Doctors Who Explain Treatment Without Big Fancy Words. Orthodontics is not a one-time-visit type of treatment. Undergoing orthodontic treatment is a long-term relationship that you (and your child) have with your doctor. Treatment can take a couple of years, and retention is for a lifetime. So, make sure that you feel confident in the orthodontist's skills, that the practice environment is one in which you and your child feel comfortable, and that the orthodontist can relate to you in language that helps you understand the plan and goals to achieve the smile you desire.

Friendly, Trained Staff. Our practice is very much a family environment, a place where relationships are established with everyone from the front desk personnel to the chair-side assistants. We want patients to see the same friendly faces when they come for a visit, and we want them to be greeted like family.

Dental assistants go through the standard training program and then come to us for additional, in-office orthodontic training at the Burrow & Welchel Training Academy. The in-office training takes several months and includes the clinical component and training on unique situations such as working with special needs patients or building rapport with every patient they see.

Clean, Modern Office. It's important to find a clean practice that uses modern technologies to provide treatment.

Modern facilities naturally equate to modern technologies and techniques. A modern orthodontist practice today uses tools for diagnosis and treatment such as:

- Digital radiography (X-rays)

- 3-D intra-oral scanning to create a model of the teeth along with software that allows for the model to be manipulated to show future movements

- Cone beam computed tomography (CBCT), which provides 3-D imaging of the teeth and the structures of the mouth

- Auxiliary appliances such as the Herbst for growth modification and temporary anchorage devices (TADs) to help with complex movements of the teeth

At Burrow & Welchel Orthodontics, we treat patients in semiprivate treatment bays that allow for interaction with other patients while ensuring personalized attention. We also offer a comfortable waiting area complete with refreshment bar for patients and family members.

A Retainer Policy. Ask about the retainer policy to determine whether it is included as part of the treatment contract, or whether there are separate charges for retainers after the braces are removed. Also ask about replacement retainers—how many, if any, are included in the cost? At Burrow & Welchel Orthodontics, one set of retainers is complimentary with treatment. Additional retainers for a patient of record are available at a significant discount. We have different retainer protocols that are prescribed by the doctor and tailored to each patient's specific needs.

The Types of Braces Offered. In addition to braces with metal brackets and wires, a modern office should offer clear alternatives for patients who want treatment that is nearly undetectable. These include clear ceramic braces made of tooth-colored brackets and clear wires, and clear, customized removable aligners such as Invisalign or 3M Clarity Aligners.

The Types of Patients Treated. Our practice is not strictly for kids and teens—we treat patients ages six to eighty. But not all orthodontists treat the full spectrum of ages, which require different treatment modalities. Treating adults, for example, can be far more complex than treating children. Moving adult teeth is a slower process, and adults tend to have more preexisting issues such as missing teeth that require workarounds. Coordinating treatment in adults more commonly involves referrals to providers from multiple disciplines.

Dental Community Connections. When choosing an orthodontist, look for one who has good relationships with others in the dental community. Those connections make for better planning and treatment, and smoother transitions between providers when multidisciplinary care is required. For instance, a patient may need jaw surgery, tooth extractions, or implants, which may require visits with specialists such as an oral surgeon, general dentist, periodontist, prosthodontist, or endodontist for the various components of their treatment plan.

Types of Conditions Treated. Look for an orthodontist who has experience in dealing with everything from Phase I and II treatments in youth to adult comprehensive treatment. Whether it's a case of mild crowding or relapsed teeth that require a multidisciplinary approach to treat, the orthodontist needs to know what you need and want from treatment.

A Community Presence. Orthodontics is about more than straightening teeth. It's about giving back in other ways beyond creating pretty smiles.

Look for a provider who knows what it means to be a member of the community as a whole. At Burrow & Welchel Orthodontics, we feel it's our responsibility to help make the community a better place for everyone. To do that, we provide financial support for area organizations and our team gets involved in monthly and quarterly events throughout the year.

ARE ALL OF YOUR TREATMENTS IN-HOUSE?

*Comprehensive care sometimes means referrals
to other providers.*

SOME ORTHODONTIC CASES can be very complex, requiring treatment from multiple providers. When that happens, we work with other providers to create a plan for treatment that includes establishing specific goals. We then help guide patients through each step of the treatment plan. For instance, if a patient needs jaw surgery to correct a bite, we start treatment by putting them in braces to straighten their teeth and get them in the proper position relative to each jaw, and then the oral surgeon positions the jaws where they need to be. After that, the braces will stay on for a few months while the jaws heal and while we complete the final details of the orthodontic treatment.

When we see issues that indicate a potential obstruction of the airway, we may send the patient to an ear, nose, and throat specialist (ENT) for an evaluation. For instance, if a young child shows signs of mouth-breathing or enlarged tonsils and adenoids, we may send them to an ENT for further evaluation. If deemed necessary by the ENT, the child may also be referred to an allergist.

We also work with pediatricians, pediatric dentists, and plastic surgeons, particularly on some of the more difficult craniofacial patients or special needs patients. In these types of patients, if treatment requires surgery, for example, we may be in attendance in the operating room to help place an appliance rather than doing the procedure in-office.

We also work hand-in-hand with periodontists, or gum specialists. Periodontists can place implants, expose impacted teeth, and monitor the health of the gums and bone throughout orthodontic treatment. The latter of these is especially important for adult patients who have a history of periodontal disease, since healthy gums and bones are crucial for moving teeth without creating long-term problems.

While many patients require only the treatments that we provide, for those who need more, it's important to note that orthodontics is not an island. When needed, we sit down with other providers to ensure a smooth transition between all the components of a treatment plan.

WHY IS YOUR TREATMENT BETTER THAN DO-IT-YOURSELF OPTIONS I CAN BUY ONLINE?

Moving teeth effectively takes more than an order through the mail.

TODAY, IT'S BECOMING popular to use do-it-yourself clear aligners that are sold online. But the problem with these products is that you're not under constant supervision of a licensed dental or orthodontic professional.

With the online options, the patient is mailed material to use in creating an impression of their teeth, or they are scheduled for a 3-D scan of their mouth with a technician in their local area. The scan of the teeth is sent off to the maker of the aligners, where a dentist or sometimes an orthodontist approves the case without having clinically evaluated the patient. The aligners are then sent to the patient, who ideally follows the treatment plan as determined by the manufacturer.

However, once the aligners are mailed to the patient, no doctor monitors the treatment from that point on. No one is there to intervene if something goes awry.

Do-it-yourself aligners do not include bonding attachments to your teeth to deal with customized or complex needs. Without attachments, teeth do not move very efficiently, so a lot of people show imperfect results because the treatment mechanics are not ideal.

Another major concern for those choosing the DIY route for orthodontic treatment is that the bite relationship can be worsened without constant supervision. Since they are only aligning teeth and not looking at the relationship of everything in the mouth, DIY aligners can actually worsen the bite in some patients. That can lead to some very bad issues such as wear on the edges of teeth, jaw pain, discomfort when chewing, and inability to chew efficiently. Simply aligning teeth without considering how the teeth fit together can be more detrimental than no treatment at all.

In fact, without a qualified provider guiding treatment, some very bad things can and have happened, including loss of teeth, particularly when the patient has undiagnosed periodontal disease before starting the aligner treatment. The aligners can potentiate bone and gum loss without proper diagnosis and literally make patients' teeth fall out. All because a qualified provider is not overseeing treatment. Plus, these companies make you sign long waivers that defer the liability for your health to you, so if something does go wrong, the patient is solely responsible—the aligner company is relieved of responsibility.

CONCLUSION—YOUR NEW SMILE

HOPEFULLY, YOU FOUND our book to be a resourceful tool to help you better understand orthodontic treatment. We want the orthodontic experience to be a smooth, pleasurable one. After all, we are changing not only how people see you from the outside, but how you see yourself from the inside. We want to give people a reason to smile more, to feel better about themselves, and to have the confidence to create a better world.

Obviously, we're not performing something as dramatic as brain surgery. But we are changing lives by creating smiles that make people more self-confident. And when your level of confidence improves, so do other areas of your life. Truly, there's more power in a smile than almost anything.

Investing in orthodontic treatment is investing in your future. There are two sides to the equation: better aesthetics and better health. The latter includes both physical and mental health, because when you look good, you feel good, too. And when you project that happiness, it comes back to you as well.

Still not convinced that orthodontic treatment is right for your issues? Then remember these key points:

- Straight teeth are easier to keep clean, and that can mean better oral health for the long term.

- Gum disease is being linked to other chronic and even debilitating diseases, including diabetes, heart disease, respiratory ailments, and even cancer.[11]

- Studies have found that orthodontics can enhance self-esteem and improve a person's social life.[12]

- Studies have also found that people with a beautiful smile are viewed as more memorable, trustworthy, smarter, employable, wealthier, successful, and more.[13]

A beautiful, healthy smile can even turn back the clock—nothing peels away the years like a broad smile of straight, white teeth.

Whether you're starting treatment or at the end of the journey, we want to congratulate you for taking the initiative in reading about orthodontics today. That's the first step in a happier, healthier future.

11   "Gum Disease and Other Systemic Diseases," American Academy of Periodontology, accessed April 10, 2018, https://www.perio.org/consumer/other-systemic-diseases.

12   John Roger Feusier, "Does orthodontic treatment in adolescents affect quality of life? A practice-based research model."

13   Sharon Jayson, "What singles want: Survey looks at attraction, turnoffs," USA Today, February 5, 2013, accessed January 11, 2018, https://www.usatoday.com/story/news/nation/2013/02/04/singles-dating-attraction-facebook/1878265.

OUR SERVICES

At Burrow & Welchel Orthodontics, we offer a full range of the most advanced braces to meet the individual needs and lifestyles of each patient. From metal braces and clear braces to Invisalign and clear aligners, we have the experience to help you achieve the smile of your dreams.

We are proud to welcome you to our practice. Here, you'll find:

- Award-winning doctors voted "Best in Charlotte"
- Over fifty years of combined experience
- Custom treatment plans for each patient
- Complimentary consultations, interest-free payment plans, flexible appointment times
- State-of-the-art facilities in three great locations

Our services include:

- **Braces**, including high-grade, stainless steel metal braces primarily for children and adolescents and clear ceramic braces, which are especially popular with teens and adults.

- **Invisalign** and 3M Clarity clear aligners that are custom made, worn day and night, and slowly move teeth into place. Today's clear aligners can treat more cases than ever before.

- **Retainers** made of wire and acrylic to help teeth settle into their new positions and keep them in place for a lifetime.

BURROW & WELCHEL ORTHODONTICS

2711 RANDOLPH RD, SUITE 600
CHARLOTTE, NC 28207
704-325-4217

1033 BAYSHORE DRIVE, SUITE B
ROCK HILL, SC 29723
803-701-9202

11010 S. TRYON STREET
CHARLOTTE, NC 28273

Printed in the USA
CPSIA information can be obtained
at www.ICGtesting.com
JSHW012034140824
68134JS00033B/3047